The authors have provided a useful and straightforward approach to dealing with the emotional distress that often accompanies cancer and its treatment. The strategies provided are grounded in good clinical science and are both practical and efficacious. The guide should be a real resource for anyone dealing with cancer.

—Steven D. Hollon, Ph.D., professor of psychology at Vanderbilt University

A Cancer Patient's Guide to Overcoming Depression and Anxiety is an excellent reference for patients, students, and clinicians alike. It provides a readable overall style and flow and captures practically relevant information that is informed by cutting-edge work in the field. Hopko and Lejuez have provided a much-needed resource to patients and scholars alike with this important and timely book.

—Michael J. Zvolensky, Ph.D., associate professor of psychology at the University of Vermont

A Cancer Patient's Guide to Overcoming Depression & Anxiety

Getting Through Treatment & Getting Back to Your Life

DEREK R. HOPKO, PH.D.
CARL W. LEJUEZ, PH.D.

New Harbinger Publications, Inc.

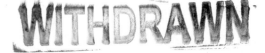

Publisher's Note

Care has been taken to confirm the accuracy of the information presented and to describe generally accepted practices. However, the authors, editors, and publisher are not responsible for errors or omissions or for any consequences from application of the information in this book and make no warranty, express or implied, with respect to the contents of the publication.

The authors, editors, and publisher have exerted every effort to ensure that any drug selection and dosage set forth in this text are in accordance with current recommendations and practice at the time of publication. However, in view of ongoing research, changes in government regulations, and the constant flow of information relating to drug therapy and drug reactions, the reader is urged to check the package insert for each drug for any change in indications and dosage and for added warnings and precautions. This is particularly important when the recommended agent is a new or infrequently employed drug.

Some drugs and medical devices presented in this publication may have Food and Drug Administration (FDA) clearance for limited use in restricted research settings. It is the responsibility of the health care provider to ascertain the FDA status of each drug or device planned for use in their clinical practice.

Distributed in Canada by Raincoast Books

Acquired by Jess O'Brien; Cover design by Amy Shoup;
Edited by Carole Honeychurch; Text design by Tracy Carlson

Library of Congress Cataloging-in-Publication Data

Hopko, Derek R.
  A cancer patient's guide to overcoming depression and anxiety : getting through treatment and getting back to your life / Derek R. Hopko and Carl W. Lejuez ; foreword by John L. Bell.
     p. cm.
  ISBN-13: 978-1-57224-504-4 (pbk. : alk. paper)
  ISBN-10: 1-57224-504-2 (pbk. : alk. paper)
  1. Cancer--Psychological aspects. 2. Behavior therapy. 3. Depression, Mental--Treatment. 4. Anxiety--Treatment. I. Lejuez, Carl W. II. Title.
RC262.H67 2007
616.99'406--dc22

                    2007036679

09 08 07

10 9 8 7 6 5 4 3 2 1

First printing

This workbook is dedicated to my parents, Richard and Charlotte. My mother bravely struggled with and overcame breast cancer. In appreciation for their tremendous support, I also dedicate it to Nicki Ford and my best friend Rick Doyle.

—DRH

To my mother, Phyllis Francin, and my two sisters, Loretta Simek and Ann Edwards

—CWL

Contents

Foreword   vii

Acknowledgments   ix

CHAPTER 1
Your Cancer Experience   1

CHAPTER 2
Recognizing Depression   29

CHAPTER 3
Recognizing Anxiety   45

CHAPTER 4
Understanding Avoidance in Your Life   65

CHAPTER 5
Behavioral Activation Treatment for Cancer (BAT-C)   81

CHAPTER 6
Treatment and Medication Management   139

CHAPTER 7

Becoming an Effective Problem Solver 145

CHAPTER 8

Getting a More Restful Night's Sleep 157

CHAPTER 9

Assertiveness and Social-Skills Training 169

CHAPTER 10

Relaxation, Mindfulness, and Self-Hypnosis 185

CHAPTER 11

Maintaining Treatment Gains and Preventing Relapse 203

Resources 219

References 221

Foreword

It is estimated that 1.4 million people in the United States will be diagnosed with some form of cancer in 2007. Everyone has a friend or family member who has been diagnosed with cancer. One of the most difficult problems confronting cancer patients is the depression and anxiety that often accompany being diagnosed and living with the illness. We are all aware of how a diagnosis of cancer can affect the health, happiness, and quality of life of the diagnosed person as well as their family members. In some cases, the depression and anxiety that occur can be extremely debilitating, pervading every aspect of the cancer patient's life—including work, family, friends, hobbies, spirituality, and so forth.

Many cancer patients and family members will address these problems by reading as much as they can, asking their doctors and nurses important questions, trying to obtain information through the Internet, and communicating with other individuals who have been diagnosed with and treated for cancer. Some individuals will also choose to use antidepressant and antianxiety medications to cope with these problems. All these strategies can be somewhat useful in reducing the anxiety and depression often associated with the cancer experience; however, the approach set forth in this workbook will help you overcome cancer-related anxiety and depression more completely and definitively, and with the acquisition of skills that will last a lifetime.

The behavioral activation treatment (BAT) approach to depression and anxiety that is presented in this workbook is a highly promising intervention that may be of great benefit to cancer patients. It can be used in addition to or instead of medications. Published research studies have provided strong initial support for BAT's effectiveness, not only in reducing depression and anxiety, but also in increasing quality of life. Readers of this workbook will identify new behavioral skills that offer the opportunity to complete the "cancer experience" in a positive way and enjoy survivorship.

Dr. Hopko and Dr. Lejuez have worked diligently to bring you this well designed and effective treatment that will teach you the skills necessary to overcome your negative emotions. As you move through this workbook, remember that there is a manageable solution to the depression and anxiety you feel. Following the recommendations of these established clinical psychologists will move you down the path toward a more fulfilling life. Overcome your depression and anxiety using BAT—as many before you have!

—John L. Bell, MD, FACS
  Director, University of Tennessee Medical Center Cancer Institute
  Chief, Division of Surgical Oncology

Acknowledgments

Development of this workbook would not have been possible without the efforts of many people. In particular, we are grateful for the work of behavioral activation researchers who are tirelessly working toward developing improved behavioral treatments for depression, anxiety, and psychological distress associated with various medical problems. Included in this list are Michael Addis, Stacey Daughters, Sona Dimidjian, Keith Dobson, David Dunner, Jackie Gollan, Steven Hollon, Mathew Jakupak, Peter Lewinsohn, Christopher Martell, Patrick Mulick, Amy Naugle, Jeffrey Porter, Adria Trotman, and the late Neil Jacobson.

No program of treatment outcome research would be manageable without the efforts of bright and highly motivated graduate students. Thank you to the graduate students who have been a part of our program of research, including Maria Armento, Marina Bornovalova, John Carvalho, Lindsey Colman, Michelle Duplinsky, Melissa Hunt, Samantha Levine, Christen Mullane, and Sarah Robertson.

We also wish to thank the National Institute of Mental Health, the National Cancer Institute, and the Susan G. Komen Breast Cancer Foundation for their support of our research.

Finally, we would like to express our appreciation for the contributions made by all individuals from New Harbinger Publications who participated in the development of this workbook.

CHAPTER 1

Your Cancer Experience

If you are reading this book, chances are that you may already know a great deal about cancer and how it works. However, there are also a significant number of cancer patients who make the decision to avoid learning about and thinking about their diagnosis. As this book progresses, we will address more specifically the concept of *avoidance*, that is, avoiding certain behaviors or thoughts, and why the human tendency to avoid can create problems. For the time being, realize that we are going to take a different path toward overcoming your anxiety and depression by approaching certain circumstances and behaviors, a process we will refer to as *activation*.

It is this mindset that will enable you to move forward in your life and to learn skills that will better allow you to cope with whatever difficult circumstances life throws in your direction. To head down this path of becoming activated, let's begin with the process of understanding the diagnosis of cancer. We'll include a time estimate for working through each chapter.

TIME: Approximately One Week

WHAT IS CANCER?

Although it may create some initial anxiety to read about cancer, the knowledge you gain may allow you to put things into a more helpful perspective and may prevent you from making faulty assumptions about yourself and your future. It may even help you and your loved ones to lead a healthier lifestyle, reducing the risk that your cancer will reoccur (if you are in remission). You may even find that some of your biggest fears are based more on a fear of the worst happening than on what is actually most likely to occur.

Even if you discover that some of your most significant fears or concerns are in fact justified or accurate, this experience may not be necessarily bad or undesirable. Instead, this will simply mean that you have become more educated about cancer. You can then process this new information and determine whether it changes how you view yourself, your values, and how you behave—and whether changes are needed in your life. If changes are desired, this self-help workbook will provide the assistance. So now, let's discuss cancer.

Statistics

Cancer is not an uncommon medical diagnosis. Men and women, people from various ethnic and cultural backgrounds, and people of all ages are susceptible to developing cancer during the course of their lifetime. The American Cancer Society (2005) has printed the following information that helps highlight the impact of cancer in our society:

The National Cancer Institute estimates that approximately ten million individuals with cancer are alive in the United States.

Each year, approximately 1 to 1.5 million new cancer cases are diagnosed.

Men may be at a slightly higher vulnerability to develop cancer.

Over a lifetime, about 45 percent of all males will develop cancer.

Over a lifetime, about 38 percent of all females will develop cancer.

The most common form of cancer in men is prostate cancer.

The most common form of cancer in women is breast cancer.

For both genders, lung, colorectal, and skin cancers are the next most common types of cancer.

Cancer is the second leading cause of death in the United States, exceeded only by heart disease.

The five-year survival rate for all cancers combined is 62 percent.

Cell Growth

Cells are the basic structural units that are essential to all living things. Each of us has trillions of cells in our bodies that allow us to function in different ways. These cells allow for breathing, digesting food, thinking, talking, walking, and many other human behaviors. Normal healthy cells generally perform all of these functions. These normal cells have the ability to reproduce themselves by dividing, a process referred to as *mitosis*. One cell will become two, two will become four, and so the story goes. This division of normal and healthy cells occurs in a regulated manner.

Throughout the body, cells continually divide and form new cells to supply the material for growth or to replace worn-out or injured cells. For example, when you cut your finger, certain cells divide rapidly until the tissue is healed and the skin is repaired. They will then go back to their normal rate of division. However, some cells may stop functioning or behaving as they should, may serve no useful purpose in the body, and may become cancerous or malignant. Cancer cells divide in a haphazard manner that is very different from the normal process. Scientists have recently made great advances toward understanding the different pathways that cells may use to become cancerous that involve different genetic alterations. Some genetic changes result in:

The speeding up of cell growth

The removal of genes that normally help to slow cell growth

Cells continuing to live even when they are damaged or deranged

Cancer cells being nourished by healthy cells and tissue

Decreased immune system functioning and inability to destroy cancer cells

So, while cells normally will replicate themselves and create identical copies, occasionally the cells make mistakes. These mistakes are caused by *mutations*. A mutation refers to any change in the DNA of a cell. Mutations may be caused by mistakes during cell division, or they may be caused by exposure to DNA-damaging agents in the environment. When mutations occur, it is common for these mutated cells to be "killed off" by healthy cells. Healthy cells have internal mechanisms in place so that mutated or dangerous cells are not allowed to completely develop.

Unfortunately, sometimes these internal mechanisms are faulty, mutated cells are not contained, and they begin to reproduce rapidly. The result is that they typically pile up into a nonstructured mass or tumor. These tumors may be benign or malignant (cancerous). Benign tumors can divide and grow out of control, just like malignant tumors. However, malignant tumors also are capable of something unique.

These cells can move to different parts of the body where they normally don't live and grow rapidly out of control. They may destroy the part of the body in which they originate and then spread to other parts where they start new growth and cause more destruction (called *metastasis*). Although benign tumors may grow quite large, they do not spread to other parts of the body. Frequently they are completely enclosed in a protective capsule of tissue and do not pose danger to human life like malignant tumors. In spite of cancer often being referred to as a single condition, it actually consists of more than a hundred different diseases. All of these diseases are characterized by uncontrolled growth and spread of abnormal cells.

It's also important to note that cancer can develop in many places in the body and may behave quite differently depending on where it began. Breast cancer, for example, has different characteristics than liver cancer. Cancer originating in one body organ takes its characteristics with it even if it spreads to another part of the body. For example, metastatic breast cancer in the liver continues to behave like breast cancer when viewed under a microscope, and it continues to look like a cancer that originated in the breast.

Cancer Staging

Staging refers to the process of describing the extent or spread of cancer from the site of origin. Staging is generally the result of a comprehensive assessment that might include a detailed medical history, physical examination, mammogram, blood tests, bone scans, or a CAT scan or MRI. The American Joint Committee on Cancer (AJCC; Singletary and Greene 2003) has established specific guidelines for a staging system. According to this system, three important elements are considered in determining your cancer stage: tumor (T), nodes (N), and metastasis (M). In each instance you are allocated a score, with lower scores suggestive of a less advanced cancer. Your T score may range from 0 to 4 and is based on the size of the tumor. Your N score may range from 0 to 3, depending on the extent to which cancer has spread to lymph nodes. A score of N0 indicates that cancer has not spread to lymph nodes while a score of N3 indicates that cancer has spread to many lymph nodes. Your M score is either 0 or 1, where M0 indicates your cancer has not metastasized to other parts of the body and M1 indicates that it has spread to other organs.

After these individual scores are formulated, they are combined to determine your stage of cancer (stage 0 to 4). Stage 0 indicates a less severe form of cancer, such as lobular carcinoma in situ or ductal carcinoma in situ (forms of breast cancer). By comparison, stage 4 cancer is the most severe stage and indicates that cancer has metastasized to other parts of the body. It is important to remember that even stage 4 cancer does not necessitate that death is soon to follow or that you're without treatment options. Every day, new and exciting developments are occurring in cancer research that are helping to treat the illness and save lives.

RISK FACTORS FOR DEVELOPING CANCER

You may be wondering why you developed cancer. You may feel anxious, depressed, scared, lonely, and even angry. The reality is that anyone can develop cancer and for a variety of different reasons. In truth, cancer researchers are aware of many factors that are linked with cancer but do not agree very much on the precise *cause* of cancer. In only a minority of cases can medical professionals actually pinpoint the exact cause of cancer. Instead, it is useful to look at specific risk factors. In general, you become more likely to develop cancer as you get older. Almost 80 percent of cancer diagnoses occur after the age of fifty-five.

Ethnicity

Ethnicity also seems to play a role in the development of cancer. For example, white women are most likely to develop breast cancer, followed by African Americans, Asian Americans, Hispanics, and Native Americans. In the case of prostate cancer, on the other hand, African Americans are at greatest risk, followed by white, Hispanic, Asian American, and Native American men.

Genetics

In addition to age and ethnicity, genetic factors definitely play a role in whether someone develops cancer. About 5 to 10 percent of cancers are believed to be hereditary in the sense that an inherited gene increases vulnerability to certain types of cancer. For example, all human beings have what are referred to as BRCA1 and BRCA2 genes. These genes are present in all cells in our body. If one of these genes has mutated, there is an increased likelihood of developing breast cancer. Instead of about a 13 percent risk of developing breast cancer (if you don't have the mutated gene), the risk extends to between 50 and 85 percent. Blood tests can be done to determine if individuals have this mutation, as well as other genetic abnormalities that may be associated with cancer.

Hormones

In addition to a genetic component, cancer may be caused by other factors that include hormones, eating habits, tobacco, chemicals, radiation, and infectious organisms. *Hormones* are active regulatory chemical substances that are formed in one part of the body (glands) and carried by the blood to other parts of the body, where the hormone will have an affect on cell functioning. Although there are many hormones in the human body, a few hormones in particular seem related to the development of cancer. These are our reproductive hormones, referred to as estrogen, progesterone, and testosterone.

All hormones are essential to human life, and all healthy cells require hormones for support. However, it has been demonstrated that cancer cells are also dependent on these hormones. For example, the longer women are exposed to hormones (estrogen and progesterone), the greater their risk of developing breast cancer. So, the risk of acquiring breast cancer increases when women begin menstruation at younger ages or stop menstruating later. The older women are when they have their first child, the greater the risk. Women who have never given birth to a child are at increased risk. Researchers also believe that the longer women breastfeed, the lower the likelihood of their getting breast cancer (Lipworth, Bailey, and Trichopoulos 2000). For men, prostate cancer is more likely to develop and grow with increased exposure to testosterone and related hormones called *androgens*. As you will see in the next section, certain cancer treatments have been developed that reduce levels of these hormones in the body and may help to kill cancer cells.

Diet

Eating habits also may play a role in the development of some forms of cancer, and it is estimated that about one-third of cancer deaths may be directly attributable to dietary factors. These factors are outlined here and in greater detail on the National Cancer Institute website (www.cancer.gov/). In particular, diets high in fat intake have been associated with breast, colon, and prostate cancer and possibly pancreatic and ovarian cancer. Although it appears that total fat intake is more important than the type of fat (saturated, polysaturated) in terms of who develops breast and colon cancer, there also are a couple of studies that indicate saturated fats may be particularly associated with breast and colon cancer risk (Howe et al. 1990; Willett et al. 1990). So what dietary behaviors are associated with reduced cancer risk or recurrence?

First, increasing dietary fiber can substantially reduce your risk of cancer, particularly colon cancer and perhaps breast, rectal, and stomach cancer (Howe et al. 1990). Second, in geographic regions where fruit and vegetable intake is highest, cancer risk is lowest. Fruits and vegetables and their associated vitamins seem important for reducing the risk of most cancers, particularly cancers of the respiratory and digestive tracts. Of the many vitamins and minerals, carotenoids and vitamins A and C may be most essential in reducing cancer risk. Foods rich in carotenoids include carrots, cantaloupe, sweet potatoes, broccoli, and spinach.

Finally, there is some indication that certain food additives or methods of preserving food (such as pickling, smoking, or curing) may be associated with some forms of cancer, particularly stomach cancer. So whether you have been diagnosed and treated for cancer, are trying to lead a healthier lifestyle to prevent cancer reoccurrence, or are simply concerned about other family members, a diet including fruits, grains, and other vegetables can go a long way toward improving both physical and mental health.

Smoking

It is probably no surprise that tobacco products increase the likelihood of developing cancer. In fact, cigarette smoking is believed to cause about one-third of cancer-related deaths and is the leading cause of lung, oral, and esophageal cancer (National Cancer Institute 2007). Amazingly, tobacco products contain thousands of chemical agents that include about seventy carcinogens, or substances that have been demonstrated as causing cancer. Included on this list are substances such as acetylene, ammonia, arsenic, carbon monoxide, methanol, and formaldehyde. Whether smoking causes cancer will depend on such factors as how long you have smoked, the number of cigarettes smoked per day, how much of the cigarette you smoke, and how deeply you inhale. Our suggestion is to not smoke at all, and if you do, please take advantage of the many treatment options that are available to you. Rate of death from cancer is double among individuals who smoke compared with those who do not (National Cancer Institute 2007).

Chemicals

A number of cancer-causing chemicals have been identified, including benzene, asbestos, lead, hexavalent chromium, chlorinated hydrocarbons, and over fifty other toxic agents (International Agency for Research of Cancer 1987). Benzene is a flammable gas that is evident in cigarette smoke whereas asbestos is common in insulation, roofing shingles, tiles, and many other products. Lead exposure also is quite common, and in years past, lead was a component of gasoline. Lead is still found in much of the house paint used prior to 1980. Tap water that runs through old lead pipes may also be contaminated with lead. Other exposures can occur through contact with various cosmetics, ceramics, and bullets. Lead exposure typically occurs by swallowing or inhaling, and although the available research is still somewhat inconclusive, lead exposure has been associated with cancers of the lung, brain, stomach, and kidneys. Finally, various other chemicals may be associated with cancer development, including less-commonly encountered herbicides such as Agent Orange (an herbicide used by the military during the Vietnam war), as well as more-frequently experienced products such as lawn pesticides and herbicides.

Although the research is highly inconclusive, there are even some data to suggest heavy exposure to fluoride in your drinking water may cause cancer. As chemicals are everywhere, including the air we breathe and the water and food we digest, completely eliminating exposure is highly unlikely. Being aware of the association of chemicals and cancer, however, can help us avoid higher risk situations.

Radiation

Both natural and human-made radiation can increase cancer risk. The most obvious source of natural radiation is the sun. Excessive and unprotected exposure to the ultraviolet (UV) radiation of the sun is considered the most significant risk factor in developing skin cancer (National Cancer Institute 2007). Skin cancer is in fact one of the most common forms of cancer in the United States, and the American Cancer Society predicts that in the next year, approximately one million Americans will be diagnosed with skin cancer, with about 6 percent being diagnosed with *melanoma*, the most deadly form of skin cancer. In addition to sun-related cosmic radiation, and less studied as it pertains to cancer, radioactive material is found naturally in the soil, water, and vegetation.

Human-made radiation can be experienced via exposure to tobacco, television, medical X-rays, and smoke detectors. Outside of tobacco, the cancer-causing effects of these objects are largely unstudied, though it seems unlikely that excessive television watching or frequent walks by your home smoke detectors would be carcinogenic! On the other hand, high doses of radiation also may be human made. For example, the radiation experienced by inhabitants of Hiroshima and Nagasaki following the dropping of atomic bombs in 1945 was associated with an increased risk of developing cancer. Similarly, experts predict that one of the long-term effects of the Chernobyl disaster will be a slightly increased rate of cancer in years to come (Cardis et al. 2006).

Viral Infection

Finally, because viruses can invade and alter the genetic material of cells, infectious organisms such as viruses may contribute to the development of some forms of cancer. For example, the hepatitis B virus is linked with liver cancer, and liver cancer is most commonly found in those countries with the highest rates of the hepatitis B virus (China, Japan). The T-cell leukemia virus, similar in many ways to the HIV virus, has been associated with Kaposi's sarcoma. In addition to Kaposi's sarcoma, the three types of cancer most often associated with viral and bacterial infections are cervical, liver, and gastric cancer (National Cancer Institute 2007). It is important to remember, however, that in most cases of viral or bacterial infection, cancer doesn't typically develop. Therefore, infection is seen as a risk factor that is likely combined in a complex manner with the other risk factors outlined in this section.

Perhaps the best way to sum things up is to say that cancer develops gradually as a result of one's environment, lifestyle, and heredity. About 80 percent of all cancers are in some way related to tobacco, dietary habits, and to a lesser degree, exposure to radiation or cancer-causing agents (carcinogens) in the environment (American Cancer Society 2006). Although many risk factors can be avoided, other (genetic) factors are unavoidable. We should be mindful of these risk factors and remember that whether we have been diagnosed and treated for cancer or whether we are free of cancer, we can further protect ourselves by avoiding these risk factors when feasible.

EXERCISE: WHERE DID YOUR CANCER COME FROM?

In this exercise, we will present you with a few questions. Please consider each question and write down your thoughts. Feel free to write in full sentences or simply jot down your thoughts. The important thing is that you get the opportunity to start thinking about these issues.

1.   Which of the factors outlined above may be most related to the development of your cancer?

   _____

   _____

   _____

2.   In moving forward, can you think of any life changes you can make to reduce your exposure to carcinogens?

   _____

   _____

   _____

3.   In making an effort to limit your future cancer risk, are there any potential obstacles or difficulties you might face in making these life changes?

   _____

   _____

   _____

CANCER TREATMENT

If you are reading this book, chances are you have either undergone treatment for cancer, are preparing to go through treatment, or have not yet decided on a treatment. In all cases, especially with respect to the last two circumstances, understanding your options and what to expect during treatment can prepare you to make informed decisions and also help you to cope with the process. Again, increased awareness can help you to overcome some feelings of anxiety and depression that you may have about acquiring cancer and being treated for the illness.

Depending on the type of cancer you have been diagnosed with, different treatment options may be more or less likely. Additionally, many individuals are likely to have been or will be involved in diagnosing and treating your cancer. In diagnosing your cancer, your primary care physician may have been very involved. A *radiologist,* who specializes in the use of diagnostic tests like mammography, ultrasound, and other types of X-rays, also probably played a role. Finally, following a *biopsy,* or removal of tissue to determine whether cancer cells are present, a *pathologist,* or person who specializes in examining tissue samples, determined whether cells were cancerous and the stage of cancer development. In treating your cancer, several other medical professionals might have been or could be involved. These include a *medical oncologist,* who will describe the process of treatment options such as chemotherapy and hormone therapy, help you decide what may work best in your situation, and provide follow-up care after your treatment. A *surgical oncologist* will be involved in conducting the biopsy, educating you about recent advances in surgical techniques, and performing the surgery to remove cancer from your body. A *radiation oncologist* may be in charge of your radiation treatments and may also educate you about this process and what to expect over time.

Depending on the type of cancer you are being treated for, a plastic surgeon may be involved with reconstructive surgery. Finally, many other important individuals will be involved with treatment, including nurses, staff, physical therapists, and mental health professionals, such as the authors of this book. In general, cancer treatment may include the following: surgery, radiation therapy, chemotherapy, hormonal therapy, and immunotherapy (American Cancer Society 2005).

Surgery

Surgery is the oldest treatment for cancer, and most individuals will undergo some type of surgery to remove cancerous tumors. There are many different kinds of surgery. *Preventive* or *prophylactic surgery* is done to remove tissue that is not yet cancerous but is at high risk for becoming malignant. Precancerous polyps might be removed in such a way, and breast mastectomy (removal) might be indicated if a woman is at particularly high risk (genetically) for acquiring breast cancer. As indicated earlier, surgery also may be conducted for diagnostic purposes, as in removing tissue through biopsy to determine whether cancerous cells are present.

Curative surgery is intended to remove malignant tumors that are isolated in specific areas of the body. This surgery often is used in conjunction with other treatments such as radiation therapy and chemotherapy to increase the likelihood of completely destroying cancerous cells.

On the other hand, *palliative surgery* is not used in a curative sense, but more to deal with complications arising from an advanced cancer. For example, in the situation of a patient with advanced metastatic cancer, if a large rectal tumor is preventing the person from being able to use the restroom, surgical procedures might be used to provide relief, though the person would not be without cancer following surgery.

Supportive surgery might be used to facilitate cancer treatment, such as the insertion of a catheter port to assist in the administration of chemotherapy. In such cases as breast reconstruction following a mastectomy, *reconstructive surgery* may be used to restore a person's appearance.

Finally, in many other circumstances, alternative forms of surgery such as *laser surgery* (cervix, larynx, rectum skin cancer), *cryosurgery* (cervix, prostate), *electrosurgery* (skin, mouth cancer), and *Mob's surgery* (skin cancer) may be indicated (American Cancer Society 2006).

Radiation Therapy

Radiation therapy (or *radiotherapy*) is an approach to treating cancer that involves the use of radiation to destroy cancer cells. Radiation therapy may involve the use of a number of radioactive elements that include cobalt, iodine, phosphorus, and cesium. During radiation therapy, radiation is directly targeted at a region of the body where cancer cells are present. A stream of high-energy waves are directed at cancer cells and have the effect of damaging their DNA so that the cells can no longer reproduce. Radiation therapy may be *external* in the sense that a machine can administer it, or *internal*, where radioactive material is implanted within or near a tumor.

If you are receiving external radiation, the typical course of treatment will be about five days per week for several weeks. Although radiotherapy is useful for destroying cancerous cells, some healthy cells can also be damaged with this process, including cells in the hair follicles and skin. This is why certain side effects of radiation therapy may occur, many of which depend on the dose and schedule of radiation. Among these side effects are hair loss, skin lesions or skin shedding, nausea, vomiting, fatigue, and increased susceptibility to infection.

Depending on the type and stage of cancer development, radiation may be the only form of treatment for your cancer or may be a component of a more comprehensive treatment that includes other interventions discussed in this section. Radiation therapy is considered an effective form of cancer intervention and has been used on a number of different cancer types, including breast cancer, colon cancer, Hodgkin's disease, kidney cancer, oral cancer, prostate cancer, and skin cancer.

Chemotherapy

Unlike surgery and radiation therapies, which are considered localized interventions, chemotherapy is a *systemic* treatment: that is, one that is used to reach all parts of the body. *Chemotherapy* is really the use of a combination of different drugs to prevent cancerous cells from returning and to destroy malignant cells that may have traveled to different parts of the body. About half of all individuals diagnosed with cancer will receive some form of chemotherapy.

Chemotherapy may be given through intravenous administration (most common), intramuscularly, or via orally ingested pills. Chemotherapy is a *cyclical* treatment, which means that individuals who undergo this therapy will have periods where they are being treated that will be followed by longer recovery periods.

The side effects of chemotherapy are in many ways similar to those of radiation therapy and include appetite loss, nausea, vomiting, hair loss, and mouth sores. Loss of fertility and thrombocytopenia (a low platelet count) also may be possible outcomes. The seriousness of side effects will depend on the type of medications used, the dosage, and the duration of treatment. The significance of these side effects usually diminishes as one moves further into the recovery period between treatments. As with radiation therapy, chemotherapy is used to treat a variety of cancer types.

Hormone Therapy

Hormone therapy is also a systemic cancer treatment that is used under certain circumstances. *Hormone therapy* for cancer should not be confused with *hormone replacement therapy* (HRT). HRT is a treatment for women going through menopause and is designed to artificially increase levels of hormones such as estrogen and progesterone. Comparatively, hormone therapy for cancer was designed to prevent cancer cells from multiplying. More specifically, it has been demonstrated that many cancer cells have hormone receptors. When hormones such as estrogen, progesterone, and testosterone bind to these cancer cells, they may actually cause cancer cells to increase at a faster rate.

As a consequence, a number of drugs have been designed, the most well known of which is tamoxifen, to block the effects of hormones (in this case estrogen) and prevent cancer cells from multiplying. Hormone therapy generally is used to treat breast cancer and prostate cancer, and the duration of treatment is usually several months but may last several years.

Hormone therapy may be a very effective intervention. For example, among women with breast cancer, those who were prescribed tamoxifen were about half as likely to experience a reoccurrence of their cancer and about 25 percent less likely to die. As with any treatment, certain side effects sometimes occur. Some research suggests that this therapy triples the risk of developing endometrial cancer and in some cases thrombophlebitis (blood clotting and increased risk of stroke; McGurk, Fallowfield, and Winters 2006).

More immediate side effects include hot flashes, vaginal discharge or dryness, and irregular menstrual cycles in pre-menopausal women. For men with prostate cancer, certain hormonal therapies may cause hot flashes, weight gain, decreased muscle strength, diminished libido (sexual energy), and in some cases impotence. There has also been concern with both breast cancer and prostate cancer patients that prolonged hormone therapy may result in the development of hormone-resistant cancer cells, indicating the importance of a more comprehensive treatment for these cancers.

Immunotherapy

Immunotherapy involves the stimulation of the immune system to both protect the body against cancer and destroy cancerous tumors. There are three general classes of immunotherapy.

First, certain proteins that are referred to as *interferons* have been demonstrated to prevent and slow cancerous tumor growth. Second, specific types of antibodies called *monoclonal antibodies* are produced in the laboratory and can be injected into patients to assist in the destruction of cancer cells. Third, although the research is very much in its infancy, cancer vaccines have been shown to improve immune system functioning and may reduce the likelihood of developing some forms of cancer (National Cancer Institute 2007). It's important to note that relative to the other four forms of cancer intervention, immunotherapy is relatively understudied. However, given the exciting new research that has been done in the areas of prostate, bladder, skin, colon, and rectal cancers, it is conceivable that immunotherapy may have much to offer cancer treatment in years to come.

WILL YOU DIE FROM CANCER?

The reality is that each year, about 600,000 people die from cancer, which amounts to approximately 1,600 people per day (American Cancer Society 2005). As mentioned earlier, cancer is the second leading cause of death in the United States. In fact, about one out of every four deaths is related to cancer. However, most people diagnosed with cancer are living five years after being diagnosed with the illness (about 64 percent), although this figure varies according to the type and stage of cancer (American Cancer Society 2005). For example, the five-year survival rate for prostate cancer and breast cancer is about 99 percent and 97 percent, respectively. By contrast, the five-year survival rate for stomach, liver, kidney, and esophageal cancers ranges from 5 to 20 percent. With regard to cancer stage, although about 50 percent of individuals diagnosed with lung cancer will live at least five years, when individuals have more advanced lung cancer that has metastasized to other parts of the body, the five-year survival rate is about 3 percent (American Cancer Society 2005).

In considering the information provided in the previous paragraphs, several issues should be considered. Because much of the information going into determining survival rates is several years old, estimates probably don't accurately reflect recent advances in cancer interventions. With medical advances, the likelihood is that current survival rates are probably somewhat higher than have been reported in the past. Also, survival rates generally can be somewhat impersonal and insensitive to your unique situation and circumstances (such as health-related behaviors, dietary habits, and alcohol and drug use).

In our experience, some people will prefer to have this information whereas others would prefer not to think about the statistics. Neither choice is necessarily right or wrong. The important thing is that you have enough information to adequately understand your diagnosis, receive adequate treatment, and learn the coping resources necessary to work through emotional experiences that are associated with having cancer.

EXERCISE: WHAT YOU'VE LEARNED ABOUT CANCER

So far, you've been exposed to quite a lot of information about cancer. Some of this material you probably already knew, and some you probably didn't.

1. What were the two most important or most interesting pieces of information you learned?

    _____

    _____

    _____

2. How does that information affect how you view cancer, the causes of cancer, and your treatment?

    _____

    _____

    _____

You have already taken your first step on the path toward overcoming your anxiety and depression by learning more about cancer. You may want even more detailed information, which can be discovered through referencing some of the organizations and resources listed in the Resources section at the back of this book. Remember, although more information initially may create more feelings of anxiety or depression, being fully informed is crucial in the pursuit of good mental health. Future chapters will teach you how to cope with some of these emotions as they come up.

THE EMOTIONAL EXPERIENCE OF DIAGNOSIS

The word "cancer" generally causes a strong physiological reaction when it is heard or spoken. Through the course of our lives, the words and sounds that we hear come to be associated with positive, negative, or neutral emotional experiences. When people hear words like "sunshine," "flower," and "beach," a positive experience generally follows. Pleasant feelings and thoughts of relaxation, comfort, happiness, and joy may follow, feelings that may be accompanied by bodily changes such as decreased heart rate, slower breathing, and diminished perspiration. Even certain sounds that we hear have a strong emotional effect.

For example, research shows us that mothers and nonmothers respond very differently to hearing the cries of an infant. Mothers, whether it's their child or someone else's, generally will experience an increased heart rate and other signs of physiological arousal when they hear a distressed infant, a reaction that isn't shared by women who are not mothers (Purhonen et al. 2001). This experience is due to a learning history in which the mother has learned that infant crying signals a need to react and behave in a way that will reduce the distress of the infant. This reaction happens virtually automatically, and as mentioned, may generalize to other infants. Indeed, words and sounds are very powerful.

Physiological, Cognitive, and Behavioral Responses to a Diagnosis of Cancer

"Cancer" is a word that has largely been associated with negative physiological, cognitive, and behavioral reactions. For example, individuals who hear that they are diagnosed with cancer may exhibit strong physical responses that include increased heart rate, difficulties breathing or hyperventilation, increased perspiration, shaking or trembling, feelings of abdominal distress and nausea, and increased production of *cortisol* (a stress hormone). Cognitive processes or the particular thoughts that are associated with being diagnosed with cancer may include fears of death and dying, concerns about the severity of the illness, feelings of unpredictability and lack of control, worries about loved ones, concerns over who will look after your children and what will happen to your job, thoughts of impending treatments and side effects, worries about whether your insurance will cover treatment, beliefs of an unjust world, and many other thoughts.

Research also shows that more generally, your attention and memory might become impaired. One interesting study even found that when women who had a family history of breast cancer were asked to read through a list of cancer-related words printed in different colors (called a *Stroop task*), they took longer to read and made more errors than women with no family history of breast cancer (Erblich et al. 2003). Thus, one could conclude that if even words associated with cancer interfered with the ability to function in a research-study experiment, then thoughts, conversations, and any other reminders of cancer could interfere dramatically with one's functioning in daily life.

Behaviorally, there also is a tremendous range of reactions in people diagnosed with cancer. Among these different reactions may be crying uncontrollably, restlessness and pacing, acting angrily and even yelling, increasing drug and alcohol intake, social isolation, foot tapping, reassurance seeking, and general efforts to avoid the idea of cancer and having to think about it by using various distraction strategies.

There also are a number of clinical professionals and researchers who consider the experience of being diagnosed with cancer to be traumatic in nature, so much so that it may cause symptoms associated with an anxiety condition referred to as post-traumatic stress disorder (PTSD; Smith et al. 1999). PTSD refers to the experience of intense fear, hopelessness, or horror resulting from an extreme traumatic event. There are three major symptom clusters associated with PTSD.

1. *Re-experiencing* refers to experiences in which the traumatized individual relives trauma through flashbacks, nightmares, memories, thoughts, and images related

to the trauma. Research suggests that between 40 to 70 percent of individuals with cancer may experience these intrusive memories or flashbacks, particularly those associated with being diagnosed with cancer or some aspect of cancer treatment (Smith et al. 1999).

2. *Avoidance* involves attempts to avoid situations that bring back memories of the trauma. A theme of this book, avoidance may involve attempts to avoid talking about cancer, learning about cancer, recalling and processing experiences of being diagnosed with and treated for cancer, and avoiding people and places (sometimes health care facilities) that remind an individual about cancer.

3. *Hyperarousal* involves symptoms that occur when some experience or event triggers memories of a trauma. These symptoms might include decreased concentration, increased alertness, a startle response, insomnia, irritability, and increased physiological responses.

Emotional Responses to Cancer

In addition to the physiological, cognitive, and behavioral consequences of being diagnosed with and living with cancer, a number of different emotions may be experienced. Many cancer patients experience feelings of anxiety, fear, disbelief, shock, and anger. They may be completely overwhelmed by the amount of information they are asked to understand about their cancer and their treatment options, as well as the many significant decisions they will have to make as they adjust to their new situation. Like any major life event, understanding that you have cancer takes time to accept. It may be important to keep in mind that as overwhelming as a cancer diagnosis may be, there are a lot of cancer survivors who point to their battle against cancer as a key element in helping them evaluate their lives and values, as well as find strengths and abilities inside themselves that they thought did not exist. Later on in this book we will explore these ideas.

ANXIETY

Anxiety is one very normal reaction to cancer. Anxiety, stress, or tension may be experienced at many different stages, including cancer assessment and diagnosis, cancer treatment, or during the post-treatment phase where one might anticipate a recurrence of cancer. At severe enough levels, anxiety can increase bodily pain, interfere with sleep, and substantially affect both the patient's and family's quality of life. Feelings of anxiety may not always be persistent and may wax and wane throughout the course of one's life.

Severity of anxiety across individuals also will vary tremendously, and many patients will be able to reduce anxiety through increased education about cancer and its treatment, as well as by learning more effective ways of coping such as those available in this book. If individuals have experienced an anxiety disorder prior to being diagnosed with cancer, they will be more vulnerable to developing anxiety during this time of increased stress.

Whether or not anxiety intensifies also will depend on degree of bodily pain, social support, and the effectiveness of cancer treatment. It's also true that certain forms of chemotherapy may worsen feelings of anxiety. Although anxiety reactions differ considerably across patients, it has been demonstrated that individuals with advanced cancer experience their most intense anxiety not due to fears of death and dying, but rather from fears of pain, social isolation, or being overly dependent on friends and family.

DEPRESSION

Depression also is highly prevalent among cancer patients, with an estimated 20 to 50 percent of cancer patients who meet criteria for clinical depression (Croyle & Rowland 2003). As with anxiety, cancer patients may develop depression at any stage during their illness and treatment. Individuals with cancer are about four times as likely to develop clinical depression relative to the rest of the population (Spiegel and Giese-Davis 2003). Cancer patients who have more severe physical disabilities and a higher cancer staging (increased severity) may be at particularly high risk for developing depression. Among cancer patients, depression also reduces quality of life, with substantial deterioration in the quality of one's recreational activities, social life, family relationships, self-care skills, physical activities, and sleep.

In addition, compared with cancer patients who aren't depressed, those who suffer from depression experience more bodily pain, more rapid progression of cancer symptoms, and increased mortality (Ciaramella and Poli 2001). It certainly is clear why the diagnosis and subsequent treatment of cancer can cause feelings of depression. However, it also is true that depression may increase one's vulnerability to cancer or a worsening of cancer symptoms.

For example, emotions like depression and anxiety are associated with increased levels of stress hormones such as cortisol. As increased levels of cortisol may weaken the body's immune system, individuals may become more susceptible to many medical problems that might include cancer. Second, depression and the passivity and problems with motivation that accompany depression may translate into a cancer patient becoming less compliant with their cancer treatment, an outcome that obviously could worsen a cancer patient's prognosis.

ANGER

A third major emotion that you may experience throughout the process of living with cancer is anger. This anger may be diffuse in the sense that it appears to be a general feeling that really has no specific target. On the other hand, anger may be directed toward yourself, perhaps for engaging in a lifestyle that may have promoted the development of cancer. Anger also may be directed toward such things as the medical community, people you depend upon, God, or problems with your living situation that may include unnecessary exposure to environment pollutants and toxins.

Anger has many significant costs, including the destruction of interpersonal relationships, the elicitation of aggressive behaviors, and multiple negative consequences with regard to the development and worsening of medical problems such as heart disease and maybe even cancer.

Accordingly, although anger is an emotion that is a natural consequence of the cancer experience, it also can be a destructive force if not addressed adequately.

Try to remember that all of these responses are completely normal. The responses people have to discovering they have cancer are tremendously varied. It's important to remember that there is no right or wrong way to experience your diagnosis. Additionally, while these reactions are often experienced when one is diagnosed with cancer, they may persist for a long period of time following the diagnosis. General cancer fears that are present during the diagnostic phase may shift into fears associated with changes in physical appearance and functioning during the treatment phase and fears of reoccurrence and disability during the survival phase.

As individuals adapt to being diagnosed and treated for cancer and experience the multitude of emotions that accompany these events, perhaps what is most important is the effort to maintain hopefulness and continue to find purpose in living. Further, having a positive attitude doesn't mean never feeling sad, stressed, uncertain, or overwhelmed. The most helpful thing to do with painful feelings is to acknowledge and deal with them. Hiding negative feelings can interfere with an your ability to feel hopeful, positive, and more in control of your life. Again, this is why a major theme of this book is the idea of approaching situations, behaviors, and events that may cause fear or anxiety.

Through embarking on this journey and eliminating the avoidant attitude and behaviors that may be part of your life, we believe the strength and motivation to overcome anxiety and depression related to cancer will be enhanced. This book will guide you through exercises to increase hope and help you discover what is important in your life. In doing so, the process of developing a more fulfilling life that is less filled with anxiety and depression will become easier. As the next step toward achieving this goal, we ask you to reflect on your experience of being diagnosed with cancer. This exercise is critical to further coming to terms with your cancer, reducing mental avoidance, and developing better mental health. Before you complete this exercise, we ask that you first sit back, find a comfortable and relaxing place, close your eyes, and as best you can, remember the day that you found out you had cancer. As you remember this time in your life, think about the following:

Where you were

Who was there

What your surroundings were like

Your physician giving you the news

The specific cognitions (thoughts) you experienced

Physiological experiences

Behavioral reactions you experienced

Specific emotions that you felt

After you have thought about this experience, please take a few minutes to write about being diagnosed with cancer. Just write about the specific day that you discovered you were ill, phrasing your work in the first person (using "I") and in the present tense (as though you had actually just heard from a medical professional that you had cancer). Please describe the event in as much detail as possible, addressing each of the bullet points above.

EXERCISE: YOUR EXPERIENCE OF BEING DIAGNOSED WITH CANCER

When you have completed the exercise, take a moment to reflect on what you have just written. What was it like to complete the exercise? What emotions did you experience? Were they unwanted? Were they unwanted but in some way helpful, healing, or therapeutic? How was it different from trying to avoid the thoughts or feelings associated with being diagnosed with cancer? Remember that it will be important to continue to expose yourself to the experience of living with cancer. In our clinical practice, the more people try to avoid their experiences associated with living with cancer (for example, their beliefs and attitudes associated with cancer or thinking about their prognosis), the more they tend to have a negative mood and a decreased quality of life. In other words, sometimes people are worse off when they fight to forget about cancer or distract themselves from thinking about it.

As an example of how this works, take a moment to consider quicksand. When someone is stuck in quicksand, they will sink faster when they fight and struggle to get out as opposed to when they remain still. So sometimes fighting, struggling with, or trying to forget or avoid thoughts of cancer isn't the best approach. Instead, accepting and understanding your illness might be a more preferred approach to gain better mental and physical health. So, as you move through the rest of this book, remember that cancer is not necessarily the most horrible life experience that you will have to endure. Instead, try to think about cancer as an experience and a challenge that you are faced with, and one that you can understand and potentially grow from.

SOCIAL SUPPORT AND YOUR CANCER EXPERIENCE

Social support refers to the people in our lives who we can rely upon and those who communicate to us that they care about, value, and/or love us. Friends, family members, neighbors, and coworkers can provide social support, both in the sense of helping us feel understood and loved, as well as providing more practical support such as assisting us with various tasks or activities. A vast amount of research suggests that social support is a critical element in experiencing life satisfaction and improving and maintaining both physical and mental health. Social support is central to helping individuals cope with difficult life events, crises and traumas, and the day-to-day experiences and stressors that we all live through.

On the other hand, there also is a lot of research indicating that a lack of social support can create mental health problems that include depression and anxiety (Klerman et al. 1984). Poor social support is experienced in many forms, including a lack of affection, understanding, or empathy, or more general feelings of not being accepted. Arguing, being frequently criticized, being let down, or being the object of unreasonable demands may also be characteristic of social negativity. So, as helpful as a strong and supportive social system can be toward improving physical and mental health, an inadequate social system can greatly worsen one's physical and psychological situation.

In fact, in a recent study of women with ovarian cancer, malignant tumor growth was fastest among women who had lower levels of social well being, less support from friends and neighbors, and more distance from friends (Lutgendorf et al. 2002). Many research studies also demonstrate that well-developed social support systems serve to increase patient hope, decrease the likelihood of developing depressive and anxiety disorders (including PTSD), and may help prevent against mortality (death; Baum and Andersen 2001).

Interestingly, there are some studies that indicate that the type of social support that is most useful may be different for men and women. Related to cancer for example, males may perceive information and education about their illness as being supportive, whereas women may perceive social support as most useful when their emotional needs are being met. In any event, the fact is that positive and rewarding social interactions help people cope with the stressful demands associated with being diagnosed and treated for cancer. Therefore, one of the main objectives of this workbook will be to assist you in establishing a meaningful and predictable social support system.

Although we'll cover this topic in detail in the behavioral activation component of this workbook, we would like you to begin thinking about the social support in your life and how the quality of your social support system may be affecting your symptoms of anxiety and depression and your ability to cope with cancer. Please complete the following exercise to better understand the current level of social support you have in your life.

EXERCISE: YOUR SOCIAL SUPPORT SYSTEM

To get the most out of social support, it is sometimes helpful to understand and be aware of the supports around you and how to best utilize these supports. Please answer the following questions to begin to maximize your social support.

Name up to five individuals from who you already are getting social support and list one way that they are supportive:

1. _____
   _____

2. _____
   _____

3. _____
   _____

4. _____
   _____

5. _____
   _____

Now list social support you are lacking and how you might go about getting that support:

_____

_____

_____

Do you think a lack of social support might be contributing to your depression and anxiety? How?

_____

_____

_____

THE PROS AND CONS OF YOUR CANCER EXPERIENCE

It probably is not difficult to think about some of the cons, or the negative consequences of being diagnosed and treated for cancer. We've already spoken about the difficult and sometimes unpredictable emotional reactions you might have experienced, including fear, panic, anxiety, sadness, despair, loneliness, depression, and anger. Sometimes you may have been unable to feel at all. This is not an uncommon reaction. As we mentioned earlier, the news that you have cancer can be traumatic in nature, so much so that you may have developed PTSD. When individuals are traumatized for whatever reason, a numbing effect may occur where you become relatively nonresponsive to people and situations in your life and find it difficult to experience or express either positive or negative emotions—or both. This feeling is normal, but it certainly indicates that treatment may be necessary for you, whether through using this book or another treatment alternative.

Second, in addition to negative emotional consequences, you may have experienced a sense of loss and change. More specifically, you may not feel as though you know who you are anymore. Your body has certainly undergone some changes, and with these changes, you may feel different about yourself, the world, and your future. Your priorities have probably changed, with certain things obtaining more meaning and other things seeming less significant.

For example, enjoyable recreational hobbies may have been replaced by frequent trips to your medical oncologist. Spending time with family and friends may be sacrificed to time spent alone, perhaps thinking obsessively about your diagnosis, treatment, or the possibly of reoccurrence if you have already undergone treatment. The world may seem like an unfair and unpredictable place. You may be expecting that more bad news is right around the corner, that hope is lost, and that more pain and hurt are inevitable. Your hopes and dreams for the future may seem altered or even insignificant. You may feel helpless, wondering how this could have happened to you in the first place. If you are spiritual, you may question your faith. Perhaps most importantly, your focus and thoughts about death and dying may be so extensive that you cannot concentrate on anything else in your life.

Third, if you are about to undergo treatment or have already completed treatment, there will be or has been a major sacrifice of time. Depending on the type of treatment you have received, certain unwanted side effects may occur or have occurred. If surgery has been performed, for example, a mastectomy, you may feel a loss of identity as a woman. Chemotherapy may have resulted in hair loss, and you may feel that the person in the mirror is someone else.

These are some of the cons of being diagnosed with cancer, and all will be acknowledged and addressed within this workbook. For now, please remember that you are not alone and that these problems can be successfully resolved.

On the other hand, we also ask you to consider whether there might be some pros associated with your cancer. Does it seem odd to think about cancer as having potential benefits? Although it may be hard to see things this way, we want to assure you that for every experience you have in life, there always will be both pros and cons. In other words, although it can be a difficult process, sometimes we need to turn lemons into lemonade! So what are the pros of having cancer?

Perhaps the most important potential benefit is the opportunity to reevaluate your life and your priorities. It's only natural that one of the consequences of developing cancer is recognition that life can be very fragile and unpredictable. Oftentimes people take things for granted, and it's only when confronted with a medical illness or other very meaningful experiences that people take inventory of where they are in their life and where they hoped they would be. So what this really is addressing is the potential discrepancy between your *perceived self* (how you currently view yourself with respect to your values, morals, and behaviors) and your *ideal self* (or the person you envisioned you would like to become).

Being diagnosed with cancer, contemplating your life situation, and thinking about issues of mortality can emphasize the importance of this distinction. Have you become the person you always aspired to become? Have you made partial progress toward developing into your ideal self? In what areas of your life are you dissatisfied? How can you better focus and commit yourself to develop into your ideal self? Which behaviors do you need to change to become that person? These questions are addressed in later chapters, and your answers to them will be a major component toward overcoming your feelings of anxiety and depression.

In addition to this opportunity for personal growth, you also have the chance to become a more resilient person. "Psychological resilience" is a term used in psychology to describe the capacity of people to cope with stress and catastrophe. It is also used to indicate a characteristic of resistance to future negative events. So in the midst of being diagnosed and treated for cancer, a tremendous opportunity also has been given to you. This opportunity comes in the form of being able to learn how to overcome difficult situations and learn coping skills that will help you in the future.

In other words, if worked through constructively, the cancer experience can serve as an immunization against future unwanted or stressful experiences. If you have been socially isolated or have not taken advantage of the opportunity to grow with family, friends, and other important prople in your life, having cancer can open some doors for you. Whether it's because being diagnosed and treated for cancer opens some doors of comunication with friends and family that previously had been closed, or it's the opportunity to develop new and meaningful relationships with other people diagnosed with cancer, your illness may allow you to create a more predictable, rewarding, and stronger social support system. The reality is that the majority of individuals with cancer will live a substantially long time following their diagnosis. Therefore, if you are interested, living through the cancer experience may give you ample opportunities to assist other people who will develop cancer in the future. Assisting them through the same difficult time you experienced may be of tremendous value to them and also may be consistent with your perceptions of your ideal self. Finally, if you are a spiritual individual, although the cancer experience will at times challenge your faith, it can also be the basis for developing a stronger relationship with your higher power. Whether you believe things happen for a reason or that it is up to you to make a reason out of what happens, seeing the positives in any situation can help you cope with the negatives. Given this information, and other possibilities you may think of, we ask you to take a few moments to highlight what you believe to be the most important pros and cons of having been diagnosed with cancer.

EXERCISE: PROS AND CONS OF CANCER

PROS: _____

_____

_____

_____

CONS: _____

_____

_____

_____

HOW CANCER HAS AFFECTED YOUR LIFE

Quality of life refers to the degree of excellence in life (or living) relative to some standard of comparison, such as the way most people in a particular society live. Quality of life may refer to many areas in one's life, including health, self-esteem, goals and values, money, work, play or recreation, learning, creativity, love, friends or friendships, relationships with children, relationships with relatives, home, and the community (Frisch 1999).

In addition to the potential impact of living with cancer on quality of life, other factors also may be important. These include the frequency and severity of other life stressors, employment status, age, sex, sexual orientation, urban or rural living environment, socioeconomic status, level of education, marital status, immigration status, culture, and access to health care. In some ways the stressors and challenges that affect the quality of life for each cancer patient are similar, such as the need to adjust to and learn about the cancer diagnosis, the process of exploring treatment options and undergoing cancer treatment, experiencing some degree of fear or anxiety about what will happen, and determining how cancer might impact your social network and employment.

However, each individual diagnosed with cancer also is unique, with different personal strengths and resources as well as unique difficulties or personal limitations. For example, where one person may have many friends and family members to lean on for support, another may have few acquaintances. A newly diagnosed cancer patient may be less fearful about the diagnosis and subsequent treatment because of going through cancer with another family member in recent years. Overall quality of life is affected by such factors.

For each person facing a cancer diagnosis, particular problems and their potential solutions may be very different. However, there is one critical recommendation that all cancer patients should follow. The most important thing to remember is that you must communicate concerns about your quality of life to the people who love you and to the members of your health care team. Your family members can serve a very valuable role in supporting you through the experience of living with cancer, but only if they are aware of the degree that you are experiencing stress or having problems.

Similarly, your health care team can provide the best available treatment only if they are made aware of your difficulties. So one of the objectives of this workbook will be to help you become more aware of your unique situation, your emotional experiences, your daily problems and stressors, and how they relate to your quality of life. Having this awareness will help you to determine which coping skills are most important for you to learn and will assist you in achieving and maintaining the highest quality of life possible while living with cancer.

Physical Concerns

When you're living with cancer, many factors may affect your quality of life in the areas we've outlined above. First, there are bound to be many physical concerns that may impact life satisfaction. People living with cancer, particularly those who are still undergoing treatment, may experience significant fatigue. Individuals may indicate they feel persistently tired, worn out, exhausted, or really slowed down. Several medical and behavioral strategies may assist in helping you feel less fatigued, and consulting medical and psychological professionals may help you to choose the best option for you.

Sexuality and fertility problems may accompany living with cancer. Whether due to decreased energy, physical changes, or psychological changes such as issues of self-esteem and potential feelings of vulnerability or worthlessness, problems with sexual intimacy and fertility sometimes arise. Increased communication with your partner and medical professionals will be vital for addressing these issues.

Poor appetite and nutritional intake before, during, and after treatment also will impact your quality of life. The authors are fully aware that some symptoms of cancer and effects of cancer treatment may greatly disturb your appetite and intake of foods (such as essential vitamins, minerals, proteins, and carbohydrates). As a result, your body's ability to heal, provide energy, and fight off infection may be greatly compromised. As a result, nutritional monitoring will be a key element to establishing and maintaining a good quality of life.

SIDE EFFECTS

Side effects of treatment are another factor that may affect your quality of life. Although side effects will differ considerably depending on the type of treatment and will not be experienced by all patients, side effects might include hair loss, mouth sores, nausea, vomiting, and sleep problems. Skin changes from radiation or taste loss from chemotherapy also might occur. Early on in the process (and ideally before treatment) these possibilities should be discussed and a game plan developed for ensuring that these factors will affect your quality of life to the least extent possible.

PAIN

Pain that is related to the treatment and recovery process may tend to hinder attempts to lead a fulfilling life. The intensity and frequency of pain experiences may vary greatly across individuals and will be dependent on the type and stage of your cancer, your present circumstances with regard to ongoing treatment, and your pain threshold or ability to tolerate pain. At this stage of research, a variety of medical and psychological interventions are available (some in this workbook) that will assist most patients who experience cancer-related pain.

Emotional Concerns

In addition to physical concerns and experiences, emotional concerns may have tremendous relevance to life satisfaction. Central to this workbook, issues of depression, anxiety, anger, and fears of cancer recurrence or death are common experiences for cancer patients. On one level, these experiences are quite normal and expected among individuals who are undergoing a diagnosis, treatment, or survival of cancer. However, by now you should be aware that if these emotional reactions occur too frequently or with too much intensity, they can be very detrimental to your well-being and can even worsen your prognosis. This is precisely why this workbook was developed—to make sure you have adequate coping skills to prevent these emotional responses from becoming completely overwhelming, further complicating your physical and mental health.

Social Concerns

Finally, social experiences may have an effect on your quality of life. Although you are the one who has been diagnosed with cancer, the one who has completed or will soon undergo cancer treatment, other people also have been affected by your illness. It may be that friends and family have been very supportive during this stressful time. It may also be true that important people in your life are having difficulty adjusting to the illness or don't know what to say or how to behave around you. Some may have odd ways of showing that they care.

For example, some spouses or partners may seem more irritable or angry than is typical. This can be a natural response to some of the frustration of not being able to help you as much as they would like. You may experience this ill-temper as anger toward you, when it might really be rage against the illness itself. Other people may contact you or visit you more regularly but avoid discussing cancer in your conversations because of their own fears or anxiety. Still other people might see you saddened but not offer sympathy, perhaps believing (maybe correctly) that you need space. In the workplace, you may notice that you're being treated differently. Coworkers may be overly helpful, or at the other extreme, employers and coworkers may doubt your ability to perform your duties. In all of these cases, it's important to be assertive about your needs, desires, and abilities.

As addressed later in this chapter and another to come, it will be critical for you to address how your social world is functioning and to clearly express your thoughts, feelings, and experiences as you progress through your illness. As you now must realize, continued social support will be critical for your ongoing mental and physical health.

So various physical, emotional, and social concerns may affect your quality of life or life satisfaction. The question then becomes, how can you live the most fulfilling life possible given your experiences with cancer? Thankfully, there are many ways of improving your quality of life. For the physical concerns, developing and maintaining a healthier lifestyle will be essential. For example, recent research indicates that cancer patients who exercise three times per week (for at least thirty minutes per session) have a vastly superior quality of life and also have mortality rates that are reduced by about 50 percent relative to those who are less physically active (Holmes et al. 2005).

Reducing alcohol and drug-related behaviors, improving your diet, maybe seeing a nutritionist, and learning pain-management strategies also may be tremendously helpful. As focused on throughout this workbook, reducing the frequency and intensity of extreme emotional experiences such as anxiety and depression and learning important coping skills also will improve your quality of life. Developing a stronger and more supportive social network will be essential as you adjust to and live with your cancer diagnosis. To get a better understanding of your current quality of life, please complete the following exercise.

EXERCISE: CANCER AND THE QUALITY OF YOUR LIFE

For each area, indicate in the space provided below how satisfied you are with this part of your life (VERY SATISFIED, SATISFIED, DISSATISFIED, STRONGLY DISSATISFIED) and develop some ideas on what you could do to make your life more fulfilling in these areas. Take your time, as this exercise will be addressed later on in this workbook.

HEALTH: _____

_____

_____

SELF-ESTEEM: _____

_____

_____

GOALS AND VALUES: _____

_____

_____

MONEY: _____

_____

_____

WORK: _____

_____

_____

PLAY OR RECREATION: _____

_____

_____

LEARNING AND CREATIVITY: _____

_____

_____

LOVE: _____

_____

_____

FRIENDS OR FRIENDSHIPS: _____

_____

_____

RELATIONSHIPS WITH CHILDREN: _____

_____

_____

RELATIONSHIPS WITH RELATIVES: _____

_____

_____

HOME LIFE: _____

_____

_____

YOUR COMMUNITY: _____

_____

_____

CHAPTER 2

Recognizing Depression

All of us have many different experiences in our lives that create emotion. Some of these experiences are very brief. For example, you may be driving on a freeway and see a certain restaurant where you and a close friend had a nice meal and a positive discussion about your families. You may hear a song on the radio and be reminded of a vacation you took several years ago. Experiences such as these provide a context where you may think positive thoughts, feel warm inside, and even smile. When you arrive at your destination, the song ends, or you become distracted for some reason, these particular emotional experiences may end until sometime in the future when you are reminded of them once again.

CHRONIC EMOTIONAL EXPERIENCES

Other emotional experiences can last much longer. For example, the joy of having a child may last years and years. The sadness of losing a loved one also may be a lengthy emotional process. In these situations, it often doesn't matter where you are, what you're doing, who is with you, or whether or not you become momentarily distracted. The reality is that these emotional experiences, positive or negative, can pervade your life. The thoughts and feelings associated with your child or your memories of your loved one may disappear for very brief periods but often not for very long.

When these more chronic emotional experiences are positive, they may have positive effects on your family and social relationships, your career, your spirituality, and your overall quality of life. When they are negative or distressing, however, these longer-term emotions may be a tremendous obstacle that seems to stand in the way of all that is important. You may be unable or unwilling to meet with friends, your relationship with your spouse may start to deteriorate, time with the children may no longer seem enjoyable, your job performance may decrease, and you may no longer engage in activities and hobbies that you used to find enjoyable. In these situations, emotional experiences are problematic in that your quality of life is impaired. You are no longer that productive, motivated, positive, peaceful, fun-loving individual that you once were. You may feel lost. You may be clinically depressed and in need of changes in your life.

As outlined by the National Coalition for Cancer Survivorship (2007), there are many such challenges for people diagnosed with cancer. These issues include being able to adapt to the personal and social consequences of cancer:

Incorporating the illness into one's self-concept and maintaining a sense of autonomy and control

Managing the physical aspects of the disease and treatment, and complying with treatment

Facing cancer-related losses such as loss of body parts or bodily functions, loss of financial security, and relationship losses

Adjusting to changes in appearance and activity level

Finding appropriate coping strategies

Maintaining or establishing intimacy and avoiding isolation

Living with uncertainty and fear of recurrence or death

Maintaining a positive outlook and the highest possible quality of life after a cancer diagnosis

Dealing with issues of mortality

Negotiating changes in interpersonal relationships, family roles, and functions

Recognizing that cancer still carries a stigma and dealing with discrimination based solely on a history of cancer

Overcoming obstacles to financial stability, job security, and insurability

In working through these challenges, certain emotional experiences such as depression and anxiety may occur. Although in many ways these emotions are expected and normal reactions to being diagnosed and living with cancer, these emotions may become debilitating and prevent you from working through these challenges in a productive manner. On the other hand, learning to overcome depression and anxiety can take you a long way toward efficiently addressing these challenges and allowing yourself to live a fulfilling life. In the next two chapters, we begin this process by helping you to become more aware of your emotional experiences and how they are related to your cancer.

DEPRESSION

Depression is, on some level, a normal human emotion that can be experienced in the form of sadness, disappointment, grief, or being down in the dumps. It's not uncommon to periodically experience these feelings, particularly if life experiences are unrewarding, stressful, negative, or aversive. However, factors such as the frequency and duration of stressful life experiences, *attribution style* (or way of interpreting events), extent of environmental rewards (or amount of pleasure we experience during our daily activities), and the availability of coping resources may greatly impact whether these normal human experiences become problematic and evolve into an overwhelming depressive disorder. In this chapter, you will learn about risk factors, causes, and symptoms of depression. You also will learn about how your symptoms of depression and cancer may be strongly related. Finally, you will be introduced to the proven methods in this book that will assist you in overcoming your depression.

Depression Risk Factors

An examination of risk factors may help to determine if you are clinically depressed. First of all, a good body of research tells us that gender seems to be associated with the development of clinical depression (Mazure and Keita 2006). In particular, women are more likely to become clinically depressed than men. There are several potential reasons why this may be true. For one thing, because of traditional gender stereotypes that suggest males "must" be strong and unexpressive emotionally, it may be that males become depressed at a rate equal to that of women but that men are simply less likely to admit to feeling depressed.

Another explanation may be that women are more frequently exposed to certain stressors than men. For example, women are more likely to be physically and sexually abused. This abuse could lead to an increased vulnerability to depression. Certain coping styles also may play a role. For example, some research has shown that women may be more likely to be interpersonally dependent on their spouse or partner (Nolen-Hoeksema and Jackson 2001). Although many women are very independent and have a lifestyle in which they experience great satisfaction in a number of different life areas (such as family, friends, work, hobbies, religion, health, and fitness), there are some women who are very dependent upon their spouse, to the extent that they may neglect these other important activities and life experiences. This tendency certainly could be associated with inappropriate interpersonal sacrifices (giving up one's identity) and subsequent depression.

Women also may be more likely to engage in more *rumination* (excessive worrying about one's distress) as opposed to being active and engaging in problem solving around negative life events or distressing situations. Finally, certain biological factors that include increased responsiveness to hormonal changes such as those associated with the menstrual cycle and postpartum period may contribute to the onset of depression.

In addition to gender, other risk factors may increase the likelihood of becoming depressed. For example, you're more likely to become depressed if you are Caucasian (white; Hopko et al. 2004). People also may be more prone to depression following a separation or divorce. Interestingly, even though women may be more focused on relationship importance and relationship development in healthy situations, if relationships are ending, women may adapt better. In many cases, men tend to be more emotionally impaired than women following divorce or separation.

Previous *depressive episodes* (having been clinically depressed in the past) or a family history of depression also will increase the likelihood of a future depressive episode (Hopko et al. 2004). Important to the readers of this workbook, poor physical health and medical illnesses such as cancer also have a strong relationship to depression (Croyle and Rowland 2003). As you will discover, the experience of being diagnosed and living with cancer may greatly predispose one to becoming distressed, not only because it is stressful, but also because of the changes in behaviors that may be associated with cancer.

In addition to the stressful experience of being diagnosed and living with cancer, other stressful life events can contribute to depression. These may include the death of a loved one, financial difficulties, unemployment or occupational problems, and hundreds of other stressful life events. Among the stressors believed to be most significant in causing psychological distress is the death of a spouse, divorce, separation, jail time or major legal problems, death of a family member, and personal injury or illness.

Importantly, even positive events such as marriage, retirement, having a child, and home relocation can be stressful, thus decreasing your psychological immunity or ability to cope with negative emotions. Many psychologists also believe that it is not so much the major stressors that occur in our lives that lead to depression, but more the constant daily hassles that we are all exposed to in life (things like traffic, conflict, job stress, or child disobedience). Finally, although major depression may develop at any age, the average age of onset is about fifteen to nineteen years in women and twenty-five to twenty-nine years for men, with the average age of onset steadily decreasing over past decades (Hopko et al. 2004). It is important to note that the earlier in life one becomes depressed, the greater the likelihood of future depressions and resistance to treatment (Hopko et al. 2004). Contrary to misconceptions, the elderly do not appear to be more susceptible to depression.

EXERCISE: YOUR RISK FACTORS FOR DEPRESSION

In the space provided below, take a moment to indicate which of the risk factors just described may be important for understanding feelings of depression that you may have.

_____

_____

_____

Causes of Depression

There are a number of different theories as to why individuals become depressed. Most of them have one thing in common: the assumption that depression can be understood according to the *diathesis-stress model*. This is just a fancy way of saying that both biological and environmental factors play a role in depression. In other words, we are born with a certain *diathesis* (or biological predisposition or vulnerability) toward developing a psychological problem such as depression, but this problem will usually not develop unless a certain threshold of environmental stress is experienced. For individuals with a stronger biological predisposition to develop depression (for instance, maybe one or both parents have been clinically depressed), less environmental stress may be necessary for depression to manifest. For those with a minimal biological predisposition (no family history of depression), higher levels of stress might be required for the onset of depression. So let's more closely examine the role of the environment and biological factors in depression.

STRESSFUL LIFE EVENTS

With regard to environment, in the previous section you already learned that the likelihood of developing depressive symptoms could be greatly increased by stressful life events. These stressful life events could occur in childhood and might include things like emotional, physical, or sexual abuse; parental neglect; being excessively criticized; inappropriate or unclear expectations; parental separation or divorce; family addiction; family conflict or violence; racism; and poverty. Parental death during childhood, long believed to predispose an individual toward depression in adulthood, has not consistently been found to be related to adult depression. Instead, parental separations that reflect or result in family discord are the types of "loss" that seem most associated with adulthood depression.

Additional life stress experienced in adulthood could further complicate the problem. Quite interestingly, depressed individuals may also create more negative life events than those not prone to depression. For example, psychologists have come to believe that depression can increase the likelihood of certain negative events (for instance, negative social interactions or work conflict) that may increase the chances that depression may persist over a longer period of time.

COGNITIVE THEORIES

As a consequence of stressful life events, certain patterns of thinking and behaving may occur that result in full-blown depression. For example, cognitive theories of depression state that depression is a natural consequence that follows from negative thoughts about the self, the world, and the future (Beck et al. 1979). There also are learned helplessness, or hopelessness, models of depression that propose vulnerability to depression comes from ways of explaining negative or unwanted events (Abramson, Metalsky, and Alloy 1989). People with this style of thinking tend to attribute negative events to causes that are *internal* (due to the person), *stable* (likely to persist over time), and *global* (applicable to many domains of the person's life).

For example, someone diagnosed with cancer might take too much responsibility and blame herself for developing the illness (internal), might believe that cancer is always going to return following treatment (stable), and might believe she is going to develop many medical problems that will be difficult to treat (global). When people develop this depressed style of thinking, negative events lead to negative expectations, a state of hopelessness, and worse symptoms of depression. It currently is believed that both genetic and environmental factors play a role in the development of this thinking style and that a lack of maternal (motherly) nurturance and acceptance and too much parental control (or unwillingness to allow children to explore) may contribute to the development of these thinking patterns (Abramson, Metalsky, and Alloy 1989).

BEHAVIORAL THEORIES

According to behavioral theories, depression results from decreased *environmental reinforcement*. In other words, an individual's life circumstances or living situation changes, along with certain behaviors, so that he or she no longer is rewarded or experiences satisfaction and fulfillment. In these situations, the healthier behaviors that you generally engage in may occur less often and come to be replaced by unhealthy behaviors that are associated with depression.

For example, when you have been diagnosed with cancer, you may feel like withdrawing socially. This avoidance of social situations may result in fewer opportunities to have rewarding social interactions and communications, which may result in increased depression and even more social isolation. In some cases of depression, people also may lack the skills necessary to obtain social satisfaction (Lewinsohn 1974). For example, socially rewarding interactions with your friends, family members, and coworkers may be less likely to occur if you do not possess the verbal (what you say) and nonverbal behaviors (things like eye contact and body posture) that are perceived as friendly by other people and are likely to be met with a smile or positive comment in return. People who have inadequate abilities to solve life's problems also would fit into this area. Finally, the more often you have punishing or hurtful life experiences, for example physical and emotional abuse, the greater the likelihood of depression.

INTERPERSONAL THEORIES

Interpersonal theories of depression are strongly rooted in the belief that relationship problems are at the core of depression (Klerman et al. 1984). Examples of relationship problems include conflict in or the ending of a marital relationship; conflict between friends, loved ones, or family members; a child going off to college; the death of someone you love; or having a good friend move to another geographical location.

In line with this theory, depression occurs because of one or more of four processes: a) *grief*, or the complicated bereavement that occurs following the death of a loved one; b) *interpersonal role disputes* in which conflicts occur with a spouse, family member, coworker, or friend; c) *role transitions*, in which changes in life status occur that affect relationships (like being diagnosed with cancer; beginning or ending a relationship; a move, promotion, or retirement; having a child; graduation); and d) *interpersonal deficits* that involve underdeveloped social skills that stand in the way of having meaningful social relationships. So, in response to these issues, it is critical that you learn to understand the relationship between your depressive symptoms and your current interpersonal relationships and then find ways to deal with the interpersonal problems so that depressive symptoms will become less significant.

BIOLOGICAL THEORIES

Finally, there are several biological theories that implicate abnormalities in *neurotransmitter* functioning (chemicals that allow information to move across brain cells, or neurons), hormonal functioning, and structural abnormalities in the brain. With regard to neurotransmitters in the brain, there is good information to suggest decreases in levels of norepinephrine and serotonin may create problems with depression (Thase et al. 1997), whereas normal concentrations of the chemicals in the brain are associated with normal mood states.

There also appear to be differences in the endocrine (or hormonal system) of depressed individuals. For example, abnormalities in thyroid activity and depletion of the hormone thyroxin relate to depressive symptoms, as do increased levels of the stress hormone cortisol, produced by the adrenal gland. In fact, we now believe that heightened levels of cortisol may be more important for understanding depression than decreased levels of serotonin.

Researchers have identified certain abnormalities in the brain structure of people who are depressed. In particular, brain regions such as the basal ganglia, the cerebellum, and the frontal lobe appear to be reduced in size in clinical depression, which could explain some of the unmotivated, lethargic, and passive behavior as well as negative thought processes often experienced by people with depression.

Prevalence and Impact of Depressive Disorders

The lifetime risk of major depressive disorder is between 10 and 25 percent for women and 5 and 12 percent for men (American Psychiatric Association 2001). There is some evidence that the incidence of depression and suicidal behavior is increasing across generations. For example, depression is now believed to be more frequent in adolescence than in adulthood (Kessler, Avenevoli, and Ries-Merikangas 2001). Within primary care medical settings, depression is possibly the most commonly experienced psychiatric problem. From 10 to 29 percent of patients in these settings have a depressive disorder, and psychologists believe that clinical depression is largely unrecognized in this context (McQuaid et al. 1999).

Episodes of major depression also are associated with some fairly substantial life problems. These problems could include worsening of medical illnesses and impaired physical health; diminished ability to concentrate, reason, and solve problems; decreased participation in pleasurable and rewarding activities; and problems with interpersonal relationships. Having an episode of depression also greatly increases the likelihood that future depressive episodes will occur. Major depression also increases vulnerability to other psychiatric problems that include anxiety disorders and alcohol abuse. The direct (health care, medication) and indirect (lost wages, absenteeism) costs of treating clinical depression also are staggering, with about four hundred to five hundred million dollars in direct costs spent annually on depression.

ARE YOU DEPRESSED?

According to the *DSM-IV-TR* (American Psychiatric Association 2001), the diagnostic manual commonly used by mental health professionals, the two primary diagnostic criteria for *major depressive disorder* (MDD) are depressed mood and loss of interest or pleasure in most activities, at least one of which must occur for a duration of at least two weeks (though maybe much longer). Secondary symptoms include significant appetite change and/or weight loss or gain, sleep disturbance, physical restlessness or possibly slowed bodily movements, fatigue or energy loss, feelings of worthlessness or guilt, attention or concentration difficulties, and recurrent thoughts of death and/or suicide. Of these diagnostic symptoms, depressed mood, appetite and sleep change (particularly decreased appetite and insomnia), loss of interest in activities, and thoughts of death are most common. Some people also may experience what are referred to as *psychotic symptoms* (hallucinations or delusions). These symptoms generally are associated with increased depression severity, longer depressive episodes, greater incapacity, and more resistance to treatment.

In contrast to MDD, another depressive disorder exists that is referred to as *dysthymia*. This condition is somewhat different in that it is more chronic in nature and involves feeling depressed for more days than not for at least two years. Dysthymia generally is characterized by fewer and less severe depressive symptoms, and symptoms such as decreased energy, suicidal thoughts and desires, concentration problems, and eating and sleeping disturbances are milder and occur less often than in people diagnosed with clinical depression. The term "double depression" has been used to refer to people who experience a major depressive episode in addition to their symptoms of dysthymia. So a person already is dysthymic, but on top of that, as the number of depressive symptoms increase, a major depression develops. Compared with people who have major depression, those with double depression may experience greater psychological distress and have more problems with anxiety and substance abuse, and they also may be less likely to experience long-term benefits from depression treatments.

EXERCISE: ARE YOU DEPRESSED?

In the space below, review the symptoms of depression, indicate whether you experience the symptom, and indicate how severe you think these symptoms are on a scale of 1 (minimal severity) to 5 (extreme severity). Then report how long (weeks) you have experienced the symptom.

Depression Symptom	Yes/No	Severity (1-5)	Length
Depressed mood	_____	_____	_____
Loss of interest in activities	_____	_____	_____
Weight loss or gain	_____	_____	_____
Appetite increase or decrease	_____	_____	_____
Sleeping difficulties	_____	_____	_____
Feeling restless or slowed down	_____	_____	_____

Decreased energy or fatigue   _____   _____   _____

Feelings of worthlessness or guilt   _____   _____   _____

Impaired concentration   _____   _____   _____

Thoughts of death or suicide   _____   _____   _____

How have the symptoms interfered with your life (such as daily activities, job, and relationships)?

_____

_____

_____

If you checked a total of five of the above symptoms with at least moderate severity (3) and indicated that these symptoms have interfered with your life for at least two weeks, you may be clinically depressed. If only three of these symptoms were checked, but they were moderately severe and have been experienced for a period of at least two years, you may be experiencing dysthymia. In either situation, this workbook will be very appropriate for you. The workbook also will be appropriate for you if you don't have quite as many symptoms, but the ones you do have are creating enough interference in your life that you would like to better learn to cope with them, be less distressed, and be more fulfilled. Regardless of the number of symptoms that you have and whether or not you officially meet diagnostic criteria for major depression, you should know several things:

> What you are experiencing is normal. A large number of individuals with cancer also have symptoms of depression.

> As you have seen, there are many risk factors and possible causes of your depressive emotions. You cannot be blamed for feeling depressed, and you are not weak or deficient because you have these feelings.

> There are many different treatment options for depressive symptoms, including well-studied cognitive-behavioral interventions focused on in this book.

> It is very possible for you to improve your mental health. It will take commitment and active participation, but you can get back to that fulfilled and healthy lifestyle you long to experience.

HOW CANCER AND DEPRESSION ARE RELATED

Let's consider how depressive symptoms and cancer may be related. It's entirely possible that depressive symptoms may be exclusively due to you being diagnosed with and living with cancer.

In other words, you may not have ever been diagnosed with depression or even had significant symptoms of depression before developing cancer. In this case, the additional stress associated with developing this medical problem may have been enough to cause the feelings of sadness, despair, hopelessness, or other symptoms that characterize depression.

It also is possible that you may have had depressive symptoms that preceded your cancer. There is some belief that depression can increase the chances that cancer will develop (Croyle and Rowland 2003). How is this possible? Well, depression affects how people behave. If individuals are depressed, they may be less likely to adhere to medical advice and attend medical appointments, perhaps for a mammography or prostate examination. Missing screening appointments could have the obvious effects of cancer going undetected and further evolving into a more threatening form. Second, recall from our earlier discussion that depression can be associated with higher levels of cortisol, a stress hormone produced by the adrenal cortex. Excessive levels of this hormone may create problems with your immune system and weaken your resistance to cancer.

For many situations in which a person has both a psychological and medical condition, it is often difficult to determine which came first. Trying to answer this question can be like trying to determine whether the chicken or the egg came first. Although recent research has begun to address these issues, it is possible that either cancer or depression developed first and equally possible that both developed independently. Regardless of the direction of causality, it is largely accepted that co-occurring psychological and medical disorders almost always have an interactive effect. This means that having both depression and cancer simultaneously may lead to a worsening of one or both these conditions (Croyle and Rowland 2003).

For example, there is reason to believe that psychological conditions such as depression may not only increase the likelihood of developing cancer but also may worsen the outcome of cancer treatment. Depression may contribute in a negative way by speeding the progression of cancer, worsening physical symptoms, and affecting cancer treatment by reducing medication adherence and attendance at chemotherapy or radiation therapy sessions, and through decreasing healthy physical activities.

In the next exercise, you should try to identify your history of depressive symptoms and how your mood may be related to your cancer diagnosis, treatment, and recovery.

EXERCISE: HOW YOUR CANCER AND DEPRESSIVE SYMPTOMS ARE RELATED

Think about times in your life when you have felt most depressed. When were these times?

_____

_____

_____

_____

Was the worst experience related to being diagnosed with or treated for cancer? (Circle one)
Yes   No

Since being diagnosed with cancer, describe your mood. In what ways is it similar to and different than your mood before your diagnosis? If you are farther along in your recovery, be sure to consider and write about how your mood may have changed throughout the period of being diagnosed with and treated for cancer. Do you think cancer caused you to become depressed?

_____

_____

_____

_____

_____

_____

_____

_____

_____

Now that you have a better idea about how your depressive symptoms and cancer may be related, let's explore the relationship between cancer and depression in a little more detail. You're already aware that about 40 to 50 percent of cancer patients may experience symptoms of depression that are severe enough to warrant some kind of psychological treatment. You should also consider the idea that it's often very hard to diagnose depression in cancer patients because many of the symptoms of depression and cancer can be very similar. For example, significant weight loss, decreased energy, fatigue, and sleep disturbances are common to both conditions.

Of course, on some level it is also very normal to experience a negative mood and decreased interest in normal activities after being diagnosed with and treated for cancer. So the question becomes one of how to best determine if someone with cancer is depressed above and beyond symptoms that may be accounted for by the medical illness itself. Recent information suggests that appetite-related symptoms (regardless of whether there is weight loss) and a decreased ability to concentrate may be most useful for diagnosing depression in cancer patients, whereas sleep disturbances and fatigue may be least useful (Spiegel and Giese-Davis 2003). Among adults older than sixty-five years of age, it also appears that increased cancer symptom severity and greater limitations in physical abilities also are associated with an increased vulnerability to depression (Croyle and Rowland 2003).

Many professionals and cancer patients also have wondered whether the location of cancer plays a role in the development of depression. The answer is that individuals with pancreatic, liver, and lung cancer, as well as those with leukemia, seem most vulnerable (Zabora et al. 2001). Even more importantly, depression, hopelessness, and a desire for a hastened death seem most apt to occur among patients who have metastatic cancer. The duration of time since diagnosis also seems to be a critical factor, with individuals who have been diagnosed with cancer within the last year more likely to have an onset of depression (Honda and Goodwin 2004). Presumably, as the initial shock wears off and individuals adjust to the news of being diagnosed with cancer and complete cancer treatment, they usually experience more acceptance and less anger and depression.

Speaking of treatment, it seems that the rate of clinical depression may be affected in part by cancer therapy. Specifically, larger quantities of chemotherapy drugs such as L-asparaginase vinblastine, interferon medications, and some steroid agents such as prednisone also may increase risk of depression.

An interesting relationship exists between the presence of pain and depression in cancer patients. On the one hand, it is believed that cancer patients who have higher levels of pain are more likely to be depressed. However, it also has been asserted that feeling depressed can increase the frequency and intensity of pain. So just as there appears to be a cyclical relationship between cancer and depression, pain and depression also seem to be interrelated in such a manner.

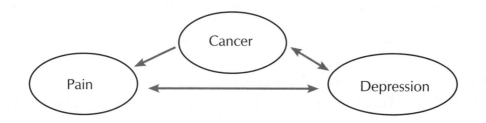

The lesson to be learned so far in this chapter is that you should be most concerned about depression if you listed risk factors in the depression risk-factors exercise, acknowledged symptoms of depression in the "Are You Depressed" exercise, have been diagnosed with cancer within the past year, have one of the cancer types highlighted above (or metastatic cancer), have pain or physical limitations, and have been using fairly large quantities of chemotherapy medications. Where there's smoke, there's usually fire. The more these symptoms and characteristics seem to describe you, the more likely it is that you may be experiencing a significant problem with depression that is in need of attention. On the other hand, be careful to remember that all of these issues need not apply to you. In fact, very few of these circumstances may characterize your experience with cancer, but you still may feel depressed. Remember that many factors go into determining whether someone is depressed, and the experience of depression can be a complicated one. For the moment, the important thing is that you are exploring these issues and using this workbook to learn a new way of living and to develop a more fulfilling lifestyle. The more you read and progress through the book, the clearer the reasons for your depressive symptoms will become.

PUTTING AN END TO YOUR DEPRESSION

This book and the interventions described were designed on the basis of a recurrent experience that we were having with our patients. In many cases, individuals in therapy, many with cancer, would present with symptoms of depression. After discussing the symptoms and life impairment associated with depression, we would question patients about how they spent their time when they felt depressed. Quite commonly, individuals would indicate that they were rather passive, lethargic, or simply not motivated to do much of anything. When asked how this passiveness might relate to feelings of depression, the overwhelming response was something like "Well, I'm sure it doesn't help to be passive, and it may make me more depressed to behave this way, but I just don't feel like doing anything." When asked when they might feel more capable of doing something, we often heard something to the effect of "When I'm feeling less depressed."

So here is the dilemma. Most people would agree that it is worthwhile to be active in this world, behaving and engaging in activities that bring about a sense of pleasure, accomplishment, and positive mood and especially behaviors that are consistent with a person's values and morals. However, a depressed individual often does not engage in such behaviors because of depression. Instead, the idea is that once the depression lifts, they can reengage in these behaviors. So the idea is that an emotion (depression) must change before behaviors can change. Based on our clinical experiences, we assert that the opposite is true. In other words, we believe that to feel differently, one must behave differently. Indeed, in our opinion it is much easier to change how you behave (what you say or do) than it is to quickly change a thought or an emotion. Remember that the problem is not that depression is something inside you that needs to go away before you behave differently and have your life back. The problem is that depression is a result of the way your life experiences and behaviors are structured.

We want to make it very clear that biological factors or chemical imbalances within your nervous system may play a role in your depression. Very interestingly, however, there are a number of important studies that have demonstrated that behavioral therapies similar to those provided in this book can actually change brain functioning and regulate brain chemicals, just like medication (Brody et al. 2001; Linden 2006). Therefore, the behavioral activation approach taken in this book will help you to reengage in your life, assist you in behaving differently to feel differently, and may have the same effect on your life that certain antidepressants would, except without those unwanted side effects that sometimes are experienced.

At this point it will be useful to address a common question. You may be thinking something like "But I *am* active, and I'm still depressed." This is entirely possible. In fact, a good number of depressed people continue to lead active lifestyles. In these circumstances, the problem is not that a person is passive, but rather that a person is engaging in activities and behaviors that are not bringing them a sense of reward, satisfaction, or fulfillment. In other words, behaviors are not eliciting a sense of purpose in life and may not be consistent with an individual's value system or beliefs about what is important in this world.

This is where behavioral activation becomes important. Behavioral activation assists in the process of monitoring and evaluating one's lifestyle and behaviors, establishing how patterns of behaving may be related to depression, determining one's unique value system, evaluating obstacles or difficulties (such as cancer) that may be preventing or affecting certain activities, then working within this framework to design a healthier, more rewarding lifestyle that allows for positive emotional experiences.

SPECIFIC STRATEGIES TO TREAT DEPRESSION

You will learn to overcome your feelings of depression and anxiety by learning a number of different skills in this workbook. Depending on your specific symptoms and your own personal preferences, you may like some skills better and find some more useful than others. Given the repertoire of skills provided, we are confident all cancer patients will benefit from this workbook, particularly those who are committed to change and a desire for a healthier quality of life.

Behavioral Activation

Behavioral activation will be the primary intervention used in this workbook. *Behavioral activation* is a progressive approach to treatment that is designed to help you increase the frequency of healthy behaviors and the pleasure that you experience from engaging in these behaviors. The process of behavioral activation involves self-discovery, helping you to learn new ways of behaving and assisting you in reducing your avoidance of situations in life that may serve to maintain your depression and anxiety. This intervention involves a self-monitoring exercise that will allow you to assess your current daily activities, orient you to the quality and quantity of your daily activities, and provide ideas about activities and behaviors that you should target during treatment. The emphasis then shifts toward asking you to complete a value assessment in which you examine a number of important life areas that include intimate, family, and peer relationships; education; employment; hobbies and recreational activities; physical/health issues; spirituality; and anxiety-eliciting situations. You will then create behavioral goals for each of these life domains, and you will progressively work toward achieving these value-based objectives for the purpose of increasing your rewarding experiences and decreasing depressive symptoms.

Problem-Solving Training

Problem-solving therapy (PST; Nezu 2004) is based on the notion that ineffective problem-solving skills may be involved in the onset and continuation of your depressive symptoms. Supported by an increasing amount of literature, the ability to effectively solve problems may help to buffer and protect you against the potential impact of negative life events or stressors, negative attributional styles (or thought patterns), and depression (Nezu 2004). With this idea in mind, and given the frequency and severity of problems that are sometimes experienced by cancer patients (Nezu et al. 1999), you will learn the five primary components of PST that will assist in improving your mood: problem orientation, problem definition and formulation, generation of alternatives, solution implementation, and verification.

Sleep Hygiene and Stimulus Control

It is well known that sleep is negatively affected in individuals who are depressed as well as those who have cancer (Anderson et al. 2003). In this workbook you will learn two methods of improving your sleep. *Sleep hygiene* is an educational strategy that teaches a variety of behaviors to improve the quality and quantity of sleep. *Stimulus-control training* involves learning skills that enable you to better arrange your lifestyle, bedroom, and sleeping routine to facilitate a more restful night's sleep.

Assertiveness and Social-Skills Training

People who are depressed are often not very assertive. They often find it difficult or too troublesome to express their thoughts, feelings, emotions, and needs in an effective and rewarding manner. People with cancer also may find it difficult to be assertive in the midst of ongoing medical issues, treatment side effects, and emotional reactions to being diagnosed with and living with cancer. However, as with behavioral activation, the process of being assertive can go a long way toward increasing the likelihood of having a fulfilling and less depressed lifestyle. Accordingly, this workbook includes a section dedicated to building assertiveness and social skills.

Progressive Muscle Relaxation

Given the strong relationship between depression and anxiety, you will also learn how to better cope with physiological anxiety through progressive muscle relaxation. This relaxation technique involves learning how to tense and relax muscle systems in the body to reduce physiological arousal in the form of increased muscle tension, respiratory rate, and heart rate. A less anxious person also is a less depressed person.

Hypnosis and Mindfulness

Cancer patients are vulnerable to depression, anxiety, and increased pain (Ciaramella and Poli 2001; Spiegel and Giese-Davis 2003). Hypnosis and mindfulness have been shown to be effective for all three problems (Baer 2003; Hawkins 2001). These strategies are helpful in reducing common symptoms of major depression such as agitation, rumination, and perceived helplessness. Hypnosis and mindfulness also may be effective in facilitating the learning of new skills such as those included in this workbook. Through learning self-hypnosis and mindfulness you will be better equipped to comprehensively address your cancer symptoms (things like pain and fatigue) and how they may relate to anxiety and depression.

MOVING FORWARD FROM DEPRESSION

You now have a very good idea about the symptoms of depression and how depression may be related to your cancer. You have just taken another important step toward learning to overcome your depressed feelings. Depression also is strongly related to another set of symptoms that is referred to as anxiety. In order to benefit most from the strategies in this workbook, it will be essential for you to also learn about the experience of anxiety and whether you need to address anxiety problems in addition to symptoms of depression. The following chapter introduces you to the concept of anxiety, outlines how depression, cancer, and anxiety are related, and provides a basis by which to learn treatment strategies to address your emotional problems.

CHAPTER 3

Recognizing Anxiety

TIME: Approximately One Week

In the previous chapter, we discussed the psychological condition of depression as well as how depression and cancer are interrelated. We discussed the importance of recognizing depression, both as a condition that is worthy of attention in its own right and as one that may compromise your physical health and ability to complete your cancer treatment. In addition to depression, people with cancer should also be aware of how problems with anxiety can affect emotional well-being, and particularly when untreated, how anxiety can negatively affect recovery from cancer.

ANXIETY AND RELATED EXPERIENCES

The terms "anxiety," "stress," "fear," and "panic" often are used interchangeably. It is true that in many ways these terms are very similar. For example, all of these labels refer to very normal human experiences that can occur under given life situations or circumstances. As we will see, all of these terms also are associated with certain behaviors, thoughts, and physical reactions. However, there also are some important differences among these concepts that are worth noting. *Anxiety* refers to apprehension that may come in the form of feeling tense or keyed up, physical changes in the body, worrying, and having a persistent but somewhat vague feeling of threat or discomfort. Like anxiety, *stress* often refers to these same experiences, but with stress, the reactions are a result of forces from the outside world (or difficult situations or encounters) that cause us to feel discomfort. It is fair to say that both anxiety and stress tend to build gradually over time, particularly if the strategies you use to cope with difficult life experiences are poor or undeveloped.

In contrast, *fear* and *panic* are generally more intense experiences that involve extremely heightened physiological symptoms such as rapid heart rate, increased respiratory rate, sweating, shaking, and so forth. A desire to flee or escape the fear- or panic-inducing situation also is quite common. Perhaps most importantly, unlike anxiety, which may develop quite gradually, fear and panic tend to be experienced very suddenly and sometimes without warning. To assist in distinguishing among these experiences, "anxiety" would be the appropriate term for a mother who is becoming progressively more tense and worried as her daughter is later and later coming home from a social function. A person who chronically worries about his or her financial circumstances or the health of a spouse also may be considerably anxious. In contrast, one is experiencing panic or fear when they suddenly contact a threatening animal, when they are awakened by the sound of glass breaking in their home, or when their heart rate and breathing suddenly escalate for no apparent reason.

The experiences of anxiety, stress, panic, and worry are normal aspects of life that can help us learn and develop as human beings. Anxiety and worry can motivate us to prepare for difficult situations or sometimes help us to better solve a problem. However, anxiety, worry, and too much stress can also create significant problems. We know that anxiety disorders are associated with about 30 percent of the total costs of mental health care in the United States, and also that people with anxiety disorders have increased levels of financial dependence, higher unemployment rates and disability payments, higher rates of substance abuse, increased risk for cardiovascular disease, and are more vulnerable to poorer outcomes if they have a medical illness such as cancer (Barlow 2002). Thus, too much anxiety and worry is not healthy.

EXERCISE: ARE YOU TOO ANXIOUS, FEARFUL, OR WORRIED?

If any of the following apply to you, your level of anxiety and worry may be too high. Put a check mark in the space next to the statement if it fits you.

You find it difficult to control or stop worrying. _____

You worry about things most people do not worry about. _____

It's very difficult to focus and concentrate. _____

Your physical reactions are too strong or unwanted (for instance, increased heart rate, shaking, difficulty breathing, muscle tension, sweating, nausea). _____

Your worries often do not help you solve a problem. _____

You avoid situations in order to limit fear or anxiety that you might experience. _____

You use alcohol or other drugs to cope with anxiety, worry, or fear. _____

You avoid doctor's appointments or other situations related to cancer (things like learning about cancer or talking about cancer). _____

You often feel restless and unable to relax. _____

You feel like you are losing control. _____

Other people have suggested you worry too much or appear anxious. _____

Take a moment to reflect on those items you checked and the experiences of anxiety, fear, and worry in your life. Do you think you're experiencing these feelings too intensely and/or too often? How has cancer contributed to feelings of anxiety, fear, and worry?

_____

_____

_____

_____

_____

_____

GETTING A GRIP ON ANXIETY SYMPTOMS

In order for you to better learn how to cope with anxiety symptoms, it is first necessary to become more aware of these symptoms and the situations in which you experience them. Emotions such as anxiety, fear, and panic are generally comprised of three types of symptoms:

Physical symptoms (how your body reacts)

Thoughts (what's going on in your mind)

Behaviors (your actions that occur along with anxiety, fear, or panic)

Physical Symptoms

When you experience some type of threat or perception of danger, your brain sends messages to a part of your peripheral nervous system called the *autonomic nervous system*, which controls involuntary actions of muscles, glands, and your heart. People differ quite substantially in terms of what they consider threatening or dangerous. When a threatening situation is encountered, a part of the autonomic nervous system called the *sympathetic nervous system* (responsible for increased arousal) may be activated. When this occurs, your body experiences what is called a "fight or flight" response. In other words, your body is physically preparing for action. When this happens, physical symptoms develop, symptoms that are problematic if they occur even when a dangerous situation is not present. In such cases, the symptoms themselves can be anxiety provoking because you don't feel in control of your body.

In the midst of a threatening or anxiety-provoking situation, the sympathetic nervous system releases chemicals called *adrenaline* and *noradrenaline*. These chemical changes produce many physical symptoms. For example, heart rate increases, breathing may become more rapid, hands and feet may become cold or tingly, sweating may occur, and you may experience dizziness, blurred vision, confusion, and a feeling that your environment is not real or is distorted in some manner. Decreased salivation and dry mouth also are common, as are potential digestive problems that might include an upset stomach, diarrhea, and nausea. Finally, because many muscle groups tense up in the course of the fight or flight response, muscle soreness, pain, trembling, and shaking also may be part of your physical response.

Once the perception of threat or danger is removed, a person *habituates* or becomes more comfortable with a situation, or the *parasympathetic nervous system* becomes activated (counters the effects of the sympathetic nervous system and reduces physical symptoms), the body generally calms down and the physical symptoms subside.

Thoughts

Thoughts refer to the mental component of the anxiety response. As your body prepares physically for threat or danger, the mind also is active. Anxious thoughts can serve a valuable function since they make us scan the environment for possible signs of threat and therefore help us to notice danger very quickly if it does exist. As with physical symptoms, however, anxiety-related thoughts can become problematic if they occur too often, you are concerned about too many little things, you can't stop the worry, or you don't end up with a solution to a problem after a period of worrying.

Your thoughts may become focused on something bad that seems about to happen (a feeling of impending doom), sometimes ignoring alternative, more productive thoughts. So really there is a major shift in attention toward the source of the threat and a belief that a terrible experience is about to happen, even when the actual likelihood of that event happening may be quite low. These negative beliefs may be so powerful that you become unable to focus and your concentration is severely disrupted. Negative thought patterns also might heighten the physical symptoms of anxiety. It is important to notice the negative thoughts associated with anxiety, fear, or panic in order to know when to utilize the strategies learned later in this workbook. The following are some of the more common themes of worry.

> Health (yours and others'). These include concerns that physical symptoms in your own body mean you are less healthy than you really are, mental pictures of sickness and disease (yours and others'), worries that others in your life will get ill, thoughts of your own inability to cope if significant others become sick, and chronic worries about your cancer returning or that family or friends may develop cancer.

> Family/friends. This category includes worries about whether you are being a good parent or friend, chronic concerns about the happiness or well-being of loved ones and friends, whether you are saying or doing the right things to others, or general safety of these people (for example, worries about car accidents or loved ones being robbed or hurt physically).

Work/school/volunteer commitments. These include chronic worries about whether all tasks are completed and on time, whether performance is at the level that's expected, and excessive concerns about making mistakes.

Finances. These concerns focus on whether you'll have enough money to pay bills each month, whether there will be enough financial support in the future, and too much attention to the economic situation of friends and relatives.

Daily events. These include thoughts about being on time, traffic, presenting a good appearance, and repairs to the house or car. This category also includes misperceptions of environmental events (for instance, "That noise means someone is breaking into my house" instead of, "It sounds like there is a squirrel in the attic" or "The wind is blowing the tree against the back window").

Aging issues. These include worries about a loss of independence, becoming a burden to others, and being alone in the future.

Behaviors

The behavioral component refers to actions that are associated with anxiety. These may include behaviors you don't do or behaviors you do too much to keep anxiety under control. Behaviors you don't do are behaviors or activities that you never do, don't do often enough, or do for an insufficient length of time because they cause too much anxiety. Many people who experience anxiety try to escape or even to completely avoid situations that create anxiety. An example of escaping is leaving a social situation as soon as experiences of anxiety or panic develop. Avoiding might be not scheduling or keeping doctor's appointments out of fear that you will receive bad news about your cancer.

The problem with escaping and avoiding is that they help to decrease anxiety and fear only in the short term. Escape and avoidance is also reinforcing (that is, doing it once makes it easy to do again), given that you don't experience the anxiety and stress that you fear. In the long term, however, your anxiety may continue to develop, possibly get worse, and may extend to more and more situations. Also, because of escape and avoidance, important tasks sometimes don't get done. For example, you may fail to solve problems. When you do nothing about possible symptoms of cancer—for instance, failing to schedule a doctor's appointment to get evaluated—you avoid facing an anxiety-producing situation and do not have to experience the anxiety associated with having to decide on a course of treatment, but your symptoms may progressively become more severe and problematic.

You also may procrastinate, or put off things that make you anxious or stressed. For example, you may refuse to balance your checkbook, schedule a follow up appointment with your oncologist, call a family member or friend who you are displeased with, or drive on the freeway. This procrastination ultimately serves to make situations much worse in the long term and does little to alleviate overall feelings of anxiety and depression.

Anxiety behaviors also may include those that occur too often or for too long a period of time. This type of behavior also may be associated with decreased anxiety in the short term but increased anxiety in the long term. Examples of things you may do too much of include checking and other repetitive behaviors. Checking behaviors occur to ensure that everything is okay, such as calling your spouse or other family member each day to be reassured that they are safe, going overboard to ensure that everything gets done on time, reading and re-reading information about a health problem you're experiencing, and repeatedly asking others for reassurance. Other repetitive behaviors might include excess smoking, drinking, substance misuse, eating, pacing, nail biting, finger tapping, and fidgeting. Take a moment to think about the unique behaviors you might exhibit when you are anxious or fearful.

In general, anxiety behaviors can be highly problematic. For example, each time you avoid or procrastinate, it becomes more difficult to tackle the problem the next time. Problems that could be solved never get addressed, things in your life never get done, and behaviors that could help alleviate feelings of anxiety or depression never get accomplished. Tendencies to avoid, escape, procrastinate, and other repetitive behaviors may keep you from doing things that are important or enjoyable in your life.

Finally, it's important to keep in mind that these three components of anxiety may occur together, in isolation, or may interact with one another to possibly intensify the experience of anxiety or fear. More often than not, when someone is anxious, they experience at least some symptoms in all three of these response systems. Importantly, symptoms in one of these areas generally magnify symptoms in another. For example, heightened physiological symptoms may cause you to worry more about what is going on in your body, which may then further intensify your physical symptoms. In another situation, increasingly worrisome thoughts and physical arousal might cause you to escape from a specific situation. The following figure illustrates how this interaction may occur.

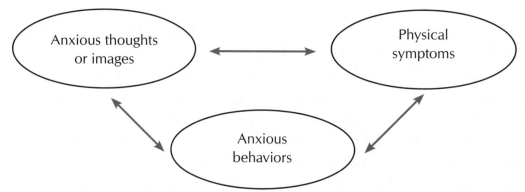

EXERCISE: LEARNING ABOUT YOUR ANXIETY RESPONSE

Take a moment to think about a recent experience of anxiety and write about the situation in the form below (where you were, who else was with you, what was going on around you, the time of day). Ideally, think of an experience related to your cancer. Then, describe the physical, thought, and behavioral components of your anxiety as just described. Before you start, make several copies of this form and try to learn more about your anxiety responses by completing this form three to four times during this next week

SITUATION: _____

_____

_____

PHYSICAL SYMPTOMS: _____

_____

_____

THOUGHTS: _____

_____

_____

BEHAVIORS: _____

_____

_____

Now, think about the cycle of your anxiety. What was the *anxiety trigger,* or the situation that began the cycle of anxiety? What was the first thing that happened in the situation? Was it a physical response? Some thought or set of thoughts that you couldn't control? A fear about the future or something bad happening? Was it checking or procrastination? In other words, how did the trigger or experience you were having develop into the anxiety episode?

_____

_____

_____

_____

_____

This is an important exercise. Learn how to be a good observer of your anxiety responses, remembering that the first step toward overcoming your anxiety is being able to recognize when it is happening.

ANXIETY RISK FACTORS

As with depression, a good body of research tells us that gender is associated with the development of various anxiety problems (Barlow 2002). For example, women are more likely to develop anxiety disorders that include generalized anxiety disorder, post-traumatic stress disorder, panic disorder, and specific phobias. Explanations for this finding are very similar to those related to the increased frequency of depressive disorders among females outlined in chapter 2. For one thing, the idea that women are more anxious may partially be an issue of gender stereotypes in which males are simply less likely to indicate problems with anxiety.

As another explanation, females may experience more negative life events during childhood and adolescence (Nolen-Hoeksema and Girgus 1994). These events may be accompanied by beliefs that the environment, world, and outcome of one's behaviors are difficult to control and predict. As with depressive disorders, this sense of uncontrollability and unpredictability may increase the risk of developing anxiety disorders. As many women also tend to ruminate or excessively worry about these negative life events or distressing situations (Nolen-Hoeksema and Jackson 2001), this tendency also may increase risk for anxiety problems. Some very important research also has indicated that, beginning in adolescence, important gender differences are already beginning to emerge that may contribute to the development of anxiety disorders. These include lower self-esteem, greater emotional reliance, more physical illness and poorer rated physical health, and less exercise reported by female adolescents (Lewinsohn et al. 1998).

Anxiety sensitivity refers to the extent to which people are fearful of expressing or developing anxiety symptoms. Compared with men, women generally tend to report higher anxiety sensitivity and more concerns over developing physical problems (Barlow 2002). Gender differences also are apparent in that, when exposed to stressful situations, women often experience more physiological arousal and catastrophic thoughts or worries relative to men (Barlow 2002). Similar to the depression literature, recent data suggest female reproductive hormones (estrogen and progesterone) and related (menstrual) cycles may play an important role in the development and continuation of anxiety disorders (Pigott 1999).

In addition to gender, other risk factors are associated with the development of anxiety disorders. One of these risk factors relates to the parenting environment in which one was raised. Children and adolescents exposed to parents who were intrusive, overcontrolling, or overprotective seem to be at greater risk for developing anxiety problems. Children of parents who overemphasized dress, grooming, and manners, or those who discouraged socializing also are vulnerable to some anxiety disorders, particularly social phobia (Bruch and Heimberg 1994).

Ethnic differences also may be important. In contrast to being more susceptible to clinical depression if you are Caucasian (white), some anxiety disorders are more common among African Americans and Hispanic Americans. These include agoraphobia (excessive fear of open spaces where help might not be available or escape might be difficult), various simple phobias (for instance, fear of enclosed spaces, animals, driving), and social phobia. On the other hand, for anxiety conditions such as panic disorder, Caucasians may be more vulnerable.

As with depressive disorders, people will be more likely to develop anxiety disorders in the midst of stressful life events. Such events would include marital conflict, separation or divorce, diminished physical health and medical illnesses that include cancer, death of friends or family members, financial or occupational problems, legal problems, and many other difficult situations and circumstances.

Finally, anxiety disorders may develop at any age, but they do appear most commonly between the ages of twenty to forty, with the prevalence and severity of anxiety disorders actually diminishing somewhat with age.

CAUSES OF ANXIETY

Understanding the symptoms and risk factors of anxiety problems is only the first step toward learning to recognize anxiety and increasing your ability to cope with it. Another important step is to understand why you became anxious in the first place. When you understand how you learned to become anxious, you have a better basis for learning how to become less so. In other words, you can learn to change your experiences and behaviors so that the anxiety that you have learned becomes unlearned. This section helps you understand how you may have learned to behave anxiously.

Learning and Modeling

Substantial work has been done to better understand how people can develop anxiety disorders (Barlow 2002; Craske 2003; Mineka and Zinbarg 1996). One of the most common explanations for how anxiety develops rests in the idea that anxiety can be learned through our daily experiences. In other words, anxiety may develop as a result of how we react when we are in certain situations. For example, if as a child you are bitten by a dog, and this experience brought about fear, negative thoughts, increased physiological arousal, and the attempt to escape, a phobia may have developed whereby you are anxious around dogs and avoid them under all circumstances. If you were told that you had cancer, an experience possibly accompanied by a rapid heartbeat, faster breathing, trembling, thoughts of dying, and poor concentration, the doctor's office, hospital, and even any information about cancer may have come to elicit a strong anxiety reaction.

Unfortunately, under these circumstances certain behavioral patterns may emerge that worsen your anxiety and prevent recovery. Specifically, your avoidance of dogs may prevent you from learning that it's generally safe to be around most dogs. Your anxiety and fear of medical settings and information may prevent you from learning as much as you can about your cancer and how it can be effectively treated. Therefore, as we will highlight in chapter 4, such avoidance patterns need to be replaced by approach behaviors that allow you to "unlearn" your fears and anxieties.

Over the past fifty years, we have learned that the development of anxiety may be more multifaceted, with many anxiety problems originating without a direct learning experience. For example, anxiety problems may develop through observing another individual behave fearfully in the presence of a feared object or situation. This process is referred to as *vicarious learning*. For example, watching another person behave fearfully in social situations may result in the development of your own social anxiety or shyness (Barlow 2002). Being with a family member or spouse when they were diagnosed with cancer may have caused your fears about cancer to evolve.

By yet a third pathway, anxiety problems may develop through receiving information, a process in which anxiety and fears are a direct consequence of hearing about the dangers of a certain object or situation (Barlow 2002). For example, a person may develop an animal phobia by reading or watching television programs about malicious dog attacks. Listening to a friend discuss his or her experience of going through cancer surgery or seeing a program on chemotherapy may elicit fears of developing cancer.

In general, there is a considerable amount of anxiety research that has supported these developmental pathways, and the belief continues to be that the direct learning experiences are more frequently reported than developing fears through observing other people or being given negative information about a situation (Barlow 2002). However, we should also keep in mind that it is very clear that these three pathways do not exclusively account for the development of anxiety problems and disorders. In fact, whether or not they actually occurred, many people cannot recall specific events that have led to their anxiety problems. It also is true that many people experience what would generally be considered a traumatic learning experience or have substantial exposure to potentially fear-inducing information and yet do not develop an anxiety problem.

For example, it would be quite reasonable for anyone diagnosed with cancer to become highly anxious upon hearing the news, with strong physiological reactions and very worrisome thoughts. More so, it would be reasonable to think that these reactions might continue for a lengthy period of time for many people. However, the reality is that people respond very differently in stressful situations. In some people, for example, these particular reactions might not be very strong or might not occur at all.

Life Events

As we pointed out in the last section, life events that involve certain learning experiences and information may contribute to the onset and persistence of anxiety problems. Whether or not anxiety problems develop out of life events may depend on many factors, such as one's *temperament*, or the manner of thinking, behaving, and reacting that is characteristic of a specific person. Past life events will also play a role. For example, if you have had previous negative experiences in a given situation or a lot of exposure to uncontrollable life events, you might be more vulnerable to anxiety. When we apply this idea to being diagnosed with cancer, a person who has previously been through a very negative experience related to another medical illness might be more susceptible to feelings of decreased control and anxiety relative to someone who has had exceptionally positive medical encounters.

Once you have encountered a stressful life event, future experiences also will partially determine whether anxiety problems develop. For example, if you first cope fairly well when you are diagnosed with cancer but then experience limited success with treatment, possible recurrence, metastasis, or a weakening of your social support system, anxiety may become more likely to develop. In addition to the role of stressful life events, biological vulnerabilities may help determine whether stressful life events evolve into anxiety disorders.

If you are biologically predisposed to develop problems with anxiety or have a family history of anxiety problems, it may take less stress and fewer negative life events for anxiety problems to emerge (Barlow 2002). So, in other words, negative life events can directly cause anxiety problems through direct learning experiences, or more indirectly by increasing stress that may weaken psychological immunity, thus setting the stage for uncomfortable and possibly debilitating experiences with anxiety.

Either a single stressful life event or multiple stressful events may elicit problems with anxiety. However, the more chronic and intense the exposure to environmental stressors and negative life events, the greater the likelihood of developing anxiety and depressive disorders (Kessler, Davis, and Kendler 1997). Indeed, a number of specific life events have been associated with the development of anxiety and depressive disorders, including being diagnosed with and living with medical problems, natural and manmade disasters, negative encounters with animals, parental death, parental divorce (prior to children turning sixteen years of age), parental mental illness, physical assaults, threats with weapons or kidnapping, witnessing the serious injury or death of another, "shock" upon hearing of a terrible event that occurred to another, rape or molestation of a friend or relative, combat in war, and many other events that affect us all in different ways.

Genetic Influences

Over the past three decades, a number of twin and family studies have attempted to identify the genetic basis of anxiety. In general, these studies suggest a strong genetic influence for anxiety disorders (Barlow 2002). Rates of anxiety disorders are higher among identical twins as compared to fraternal twins and are about three to four times more common in relatives of people with anxiety disorders compared to relatives of those without anxiety disorders.

Although very compelling evidence has been compiled to suggest a genetic basis for anxiety disorders, as highlighted in previous sections, environmental factors also are very significant. It is important to note that the role of genetic factors may be more or less important, depending on the type of anxiety disorder. For example, a genetic basis for panic disorder and obsessive-compulsive disorder is more supported than a genetic basis for generalized anxiety disorder and post-traumatic stress disorder (Barlow 2002).

Many neuroimaging studies have been conducted to look at brain functioning in people with anxiety problems. These studies have included many different methods such as positron emission tomography (PET), magnetic resonance imaging (MRI), functional magnetic resonance imaging (MRI), and single photon emission computed tomography (SPECT). Some interesting differences have been found between people with and without anxiety problems. For example, among people with anxiety disorders, some studies have found increased activation in certain areas of the brain, suggesting that these parts of the brain may play a key role in the development and persistence of anxiety.

The most important structure may be the *amygdala*, an almond-shaped structure deep within the brain. The amygdala appears to serve as a communications hub between parts of the brain that process incoming sensory signals and the parts that interpret them. The amygdala is capable of signaling that a threat is present and may trigger an anxiety or fear response that includes physical, cognitive, and behavioral symptoms. Emotional memories stored in the central part of the amygdala also may play an important role in phobic disorders, while it is possible that different parts of the amygdala may be involved in other forms of anxiety (Barlow 2002).

Finally, it is quite evident that certain neurotransmitters and hormones are associated with anxiety problems. In particular, decreased levels of serotonin and norepinephrine have been implicated in both anxiety and depressive disorders. Similarly, people with anxiety and depressive problems also tend to produce higher than normal levels of the stress hormone cortisol (Barlow 2002).

EXERCISE: YOUR RISK FACTORS AND CAUSES OF ANXIETY

In the space provided below, take a moment to indicate which anxiety risk factors you may have. Also highlight whether you believe some of the causes of anxiety may be relevant to you and your anxiety symptoms. Have you had potentially significant learning experiences that may have contributed to anxiety? Negative life events? Do you have a family history of anxiety?

_____

_____

_____

_____

_____

_____

ARE YOU ANXIOUS? DIFFERENT TYPES OF ANXIETY DISORDERS

Up to this point, we have discussed anxiety broadly. Although it's useful to understand the common features of anxiety, it also is valuable to be knowledgeable about specific anxiety conditions and how these may differ in important ways. According to the *Diagnostic Statistical Manual of Mental Disorders* (American Psychiatric Association 2000), there are twelve different anxiety disorders. Here we review six that are most clearly related to cancer.

Specific Phobia

A *specific phobia* is a strong and persistent fear of an object or situation that far exceeds the reaction of most people and creates significant distress or impairment in life functioning. People with specific phobias experience substantial anxiety when in the presence of, or even anticipating, a particular object or situation. People with specific phobias can fear many situations, including various animals, storms, heights, water, elevators, enclosed places, driving, flying, and so forth. In fact, there are hundreds of different phobias.

Applied to cancer, people may develop a specific phobia to medical procedures used to treat cancer, such as chemotherapy and radiation therapy. These forms of treatment may be viewed as invasive, unwanted, and may provoke an intense anxiety response and even avoidance of the treatment itself. For people not diagnosed with cancer, particularly family members and close friends of people diagnosed with cancer, cancer phobia or carcinophobia may develop. *Carcinophobia* refers to the experience of intense anxiety and dread related to the idea that one may develop cancer. Cancer phobia, unlike many other phobias, normally appears in adulthood and can also include a fear of death. Cancer patients also may fear needles or small spaces and may avoid having tests in confined spaces such as scanning machines (like an MRI).

Social Phobia

Social phobia refers to the experience of intense anxiety when exposed to social situations. If you are socially phobic, you may try to avoid social situations entirely. Or if you do approach these situations, you may experience extreme distress until the interaction is over. Strong physiological symptoms, negative thoughts, and fears of doing something humiliating or embarrassing are also common. Even when people with social phobia manage to confront their fear, they usually feel very anxious before the event/outing, feel intensely uncomfortable throughout the experience, and have lingering unpleasant feelings afterward. Social phobia frequently occurs with public speaking, meeting people, dealing with authority figures, eating in public, and using public restrooms.

Applied to cancer, people may develop symptoms of social phobia as a consequence of illness-related experiences. For example, social phobia may be linked to receiving a mastectomy for breast cancer, fears associated with treatment for bladder cancer and colorectal cancer, and also as a consequence of side effects of chemotherapy such as hair loss and dry skin. Because of the anxiety that often is associated with being diagnosed with cancer, and the fact that a doctor and other medical personnel often are involved in the diagnostic process, this learning experience can cause you to associate anxiety with people, a reaction that could extend beyond medical personnel to many people in your life.

Post-Traumatic Stress Disorder (PTSD)

Post-traumatic stress disorder refers to the development of traumatic symptoms following exposure to an extremely stressful event. This event typically involves actual or threatened death or serious injury or a threat to the physical integrity of an individual. The person's response to this event generally involves extreme fear, helplessness, or horror. As discussed in chapter 1, people with PTSD often avoid situations related to the event, reexperience the event (for example, through nightmares and flashbacks), and experience intense physical arousal.

Although people commonly think of PTSD as being related to assault, rape, combat, natural disasters, and similar experiences, PTSD also is related to cancer. Many cancer experiences can represent the traumatic event that elicits PTSD symptoms, including the actual diagnosis, aspects of the treatment process, information given about recurrence, negative test results, and other aspects of the cancer experience. In a fairly recent study that looked at the physiological reactions of breast cancer patients when they developed a personal narrative (story) describing their most stressful experiences with breast cancer, they exhibited heightened physical responses that were very similar to PTSD patients who had experienced other traumas unrelated to cancer (Kangas, Henry, and Bryant 2002).

Generalized Anxiety Disorder (GAD)

Generalized anxiety disorder is a disorder of chronic worry. GAD involves excessive anxiety and worry that has occurred for more days than not for at least six months, with the worry being associated with a number of life areas (for example, health, relationships, finances, employment, community and world events, and so forth). Moreover, the worry is very difficult to control, and it's often accompanied by feelings of restlessness, difficulty concentrating, muscle tension, fatigue, sleep disturbance, and irritability.

GAD may occur among cancer patients. For example, patients with supportive family and friends may come to develop fears that nobody will be willing or able to provide them with the care and support they need throughout their experience. Patients may worry excessively about being unable to pay for their treatment, even though they have adequate financial resources and insurance. They may worry that they'll lose their job due to time spent in treatment and recovery. Following treatment, they may greatly fear that their cancer will return or that a loved one may develop cancer.

Panic Disorder

Panic disorder is characterized by intense episodes of anxiety that involve strong physiological and cognitive symptoms, including rapid heart rate, hyperventilation, sweating, trembling, feelings of choking, nausea, and fears that you are losing control or dying. These attacks appear to come out of the blue, and the sufferer usually has persistent fears about having another attack. Panic disorder often is accompanied by *agoraphobia*, or anxiety about being in places where help might be unavailable or escape might be difficult (such as being in a crowd, shopping mall, airplane, bus, or restaurant).

Although it is reasonable to think that experiences of panic may be associated with a cancer diagnosis and treatment, the reality is that only limited work has focused on studying the relation of cancer and panic. Many medical and psychiatric professionals believe that when panic disorder coexists with cancer, it generally precedes the cancer diagnosis. There are some researchers, however, who report a much-higher-than-normal rate of panic disorder in cancer patients, with as many as 20 percent of cancer patients experiencing panic attacks (Slaughter et al. 2000). Problematically, these experiences with panic may result in the decision of cancer patients to stop involvement with chemotherapy. Accordingly, in an effort to ensure that patients follow through on their treatment, a great deal more work is needed to further clarify the relationship between panic and cancer.

Obsessive-Compulsive Disorder

Obsessive-compulsive disorder is characterized by persistent thoughts, ideas, or images (*obsessions*) and by repetitive, purposeful, and intentional behaviors (*compulsions*) that a person engages in to manage distress. To be considered a disorder, obsessive thoughts and compulsive behaviors must be time consuming and must also significantly interfere with a person's ability to function in employment, academic, or social situations.

Cancer patients with obsessive-compulsive disorder may engage in compulsive behaviors such as hand washing, checking, or counting to such a degree that compliance with cancer treatment becomes a secondary objective. For some patients, what starts out as normal worry about their cancer diagnosis, treatment, and prognosis can develop into a full-blown obsessive-compulsive disorder that can be very time consuming and disabling. Please note, however, that this form of anxiety is apparently very rare in cancer patients who do not already have a history of obsessive and compulsive behaviors. In other words, there is little evidence to support the idea that developing cancer somehow predisposes one to become obsessive-compulsive.

EXERCISE: DO THESE DISORDERS APPLY TO YOU?

Of the anxiety disorders just discussed, do any seem to apply to you? When did the condition start? Did symptoms develop before or after your diagnosis and treatment for cancer? What have you done to try to work through or cope with your anxiety? Have these efforts been useful?

_____

_____

_____

_____

_____

_____

PREVALENCE AND IMPACT OF ANXIETY DISORDERS

Among younger and older adults, in any given year, between 2 and 19 percent of people have an anxiety disorder (Flint 1994; Kessler et al. 1994). The likelihood of developing any anxiety disorder over the course of your lifetime is about 19 percent (almost one in five), with the likelihood of developing specific anxiety disorders as follows: panic disorder (2 percent), obsessive-compulsive disorder (2 percent), generalized anxiety disorder (4 percent), PTSD (5 percent), specific phobias (7 percent), and social phobia (11 percent). Interestingly, the likelihood of developing anxiety disorders in older adulthood (age sixty-five or better) is higher than the likelihood of developing other psychiatric problems such as major depression and severe cognitive impairment (Hopko and Stanley 2003; Sheikh 1992). Of course, as we mentioned earlier, many risk factors that include medical illnesses such as cancer may increase the likelihood of developing emotional problems.

Among people diagnosed with cancer, the first six months after being diagnosed appears to be a critical time period for determining whether or not an anxiety disorder develops. Research indicates that between 25 and 50 percent of people diagnosed with cancer will develop an anxiety disorder in the first six months following diagnosis (Kangas, Henry, and Bryant 2005). Of the anxiety disorders, PTSD and generalized anxiety disorder seem most likely to emerge during this period. Further magnifying the problem, about 20 to 30 percent of people diagnosed with cancer also will develop clinical depression within the first six months following a cancer diagnosis.

There are a number of additional variables that influence how well you adjust to a cancer diagnosis and how you function psychologically in the months and years following the diagnosis. You are more likely to have adapted better to living with cancer and are less likely to have significant psychological distress (anxiety and depression) if the following apply to you (Kangas, Henry, and Bryant 2005):

> You are married.
>
> You are older (increased age is associated with better coping).
>
> You have an adequate number of family members and relatives in your community.
>
> You attend church or have other spiritual commitments.
>
> You do not have a past history of substance abuse, clinical depression, or anxiety.
>
> You have few if any other major medical problems.
>
> Your employment and financial situation is stable.
>
> You are actively engaged in life experiences that bring you pleasure or satisfaction.
>
> You have adequate medical insurance.
>
> You are educated.
>
> You have a less severe cancer stage (see chapter 1).

These psychosocial variables can help to buffer the stress associated with being diagnosed with and living through the cancer experience. However, if several of these variables do not characterize your life, you may have more difficulties than others when it comes to adapting to life stressors and may be more prone to anxiety disorders.

If you do develop an anxiety disorder, its impact on your life functioning can be quite significant. For example, anxiety disorders have been associated with decreased quality of life, work productivity, and financial status, as well as increased use and higher costs of health care services (Barlow 2002; Hopko and Stanley 2003). Moreover, adults with anxiety symptoms and disorders report decreased physical activities and poorer physical health, decreased life satisfaction, and increased loneliness (Barlow 2002). Heightened anxiety symptoms also may increase the risk of developing or worsening medical problems such as cancer and coronary heart disease and may increase use of pain-relieving medication (Kawachi et al. 1994; Spiegel and Giese-Davis 2003; Taenzer, Melzack, and Jeans 1986).

HOW CANCER AND ANXIETY ARE RELATED

Although we have focused a lot on the concept of anxiety and some of the anxiety disorders that may be linked with a cancer diagnosis, we also want to make sure to emphasize that anxiety is a very normal reaction to cancer. Anxiety may be more or less of a problem during different stages of life with cancer. For example, you may experience anxiety while undergoing a cancer screening test, waiting for laboratory or testing results, receiving a cancer diagnosis, undergoing the various forms of cancer treatment, or anticipating a recurrence of cancer. You may become more anxious as cancer spreads or treatment becomes more intense but may be much less anxious following the termination of radiation treatments or chemotherapy. Contrary to what many people believe, in our clinical experience, patients who have an advanced form of cancer generally do not experience anxiety in the form of fears of death or dying but more commonly from fear of uncontrollable pain, feelings of isolation, or fears of having to be overly dependent on others.

It is important to mention that more intense anxiety associated with cancer treatment is likely to occur among people who have a history of anxiety disorders and patients who experience intense anxiety at the time of their cancer diagnosis. Anxiety also may be more common in patients who have severe pain or a disability, have a limited social network, or have cancer that is not responding to treatment. Importantly, cancer that occurs (or spreads) to the lungs or the central nervous system (brain and spinal cord) may create physical problems that can cause or aggravate anxiety. Many cancer medications and treatments can worsen feelings of anxiety. The important message here—and consistent with the idea that people experience different forms of anxiety symptoms (physical, cognitive, behavioral)—is that the experience of anxiety, the situations that elicit anxiety, the environmental buffers against anxiety, and coping mechanisms to combat anxiety will be very different across cancer patients.

The relationship between anxiety and cancer also is interesting in that anxiety problems may be present before you are diagnosed with cancer, may or may not worsen following the diagnosis of cancer, may not have developed until after you were diagnosed with cancer, and may or may not be associated with depressive symptoms. For some patients, particularly those who experienced intense anxiety prior to their cancer diagnosis, anxiety may become completely overwhelming and, like clinical depression, may interfere with the process of being treated for cancer. Ultimately, we know that cancer patients who are most anxious are also more likely to report feelings of pain, sleep problems, symptoms of nausea and vomiting, poorer social relationships, and decreased quality of life (Ciaramella and Poli 2001). If left untreated, severe anxiety may even shorten a patient's life (Spiegel and Giese-Davis 2003). Therefore, as with problematic symptoms of depression, there is a clear need to diminish the considerable problems that anxiety can create in your life.

EXERCISE: HOW YOUR CANCER AND ANXIETY SYMPTOMS ARE RELATED

Think about times in your life when you have felt most anxious. When were these times? Are they similar to the times in your life when you felt most depressed (see exercise from chapter 2)?

_____

_____

_____

_____

_____

Were the worst experiences related to being diagnosed or treated for cancer? (Circle one)   Yes   No

Since being diagnosed with cancer, describe your level of anxiety. In what ways is it similar to and different than your anxiety before your diagnosis? If you are farther along in recovery, be sure to consider and write about how your level of anxiety may have changed throughout the period of being diagnosed with and treated for cancer. Do you think cancer caused you to become anxious?

_____

_____

_____

_____

_____

ANXIETY AND DEPRESSION: DIFFERENT BUT RELATED CONDITIONS

Up until this point we have been discussing the emotions of depression and anxiety as though they are two very different experiences. In some ways, they are distinguishable emotional reactions. People with anxiety disorders can sometimes be distinguished from depressed people on the basis of certain symptoms. For example, researcher David Barlow has indicated that almost all depressed patients are anxious, but that not all anxious patients are depressed (2002). Furthermore, when people develop both anxiety and depressive problems, there is a general belief that anxiety problems tend to emerge first. As far as specific symptoms are concerned, it appears as though depressive symptoms that include *anhedonia*, defined as a loss of pleasure in typically enjoyable or rewarding activities, and cognitive and motor "slowing" may be unique to depressed patients. In other words, in addition to the experience of negative moods that seem to be characteristic of both anxiety and mood disorders, depressed people may experience more in the way of low positive affect (or mood) compared with anxious people. Although there has been some discussion about this issue in recent years, it is generally believed that physiological arousal, in the form of symptoms described earlier in the chapter, are more common to anxiety disorders when compared to depressive disorders.

However, the similarities among anxiety and depressive disorders far outweigh their differences. In fact, the similarities are so strong, and the overlap so high among these disorders (about 50 percent of people with depression have anxiety and vice versa) that some experts in emotional disorders are convinced that it is more useful to refer to these problems as a mixed anxiety-depression syndrome rather than as separate disorders (Zinbarg and Barlow 1991).

For one thing, both conditions seem to share similar neurobiological processes. The *limbic system*, or the emotional control center of the brain, is involved with both anxiety and depressive symptoms. Both anxiety and depression also seem to involve problems with two chemicals found in the brain, serotonin and norepinephrine. For both conditions, levels of these neurotransmitters appear somewhat lower than normal. That is why similar medications that target these chemicals are used to treat both anxiety and depression, and why these medications often are effective for either condition.

In addition, there are many similar symptoms shared among anxiety and depressive disorders. These include difficulties concentrating, sleep difficulties, irritability, appetite changes, perceptions that life is unpredictable and out of control, and even feelings of hopelessness and despair. As you may recall from this chapter and chapter 2, certain stressful life events are related to the onset of both anxiety and depressive disorders. At this stage of research, it appears that similar life stressors may be related to the likelihood of developing both anxiety and depression (Kessler et al. 1997). Accordingly, it seems as though many people may be biologically prone to develop problems with anxiety and depression, and, especially if they have had life experiences that involve a lack of control or unpredictability and have experienced significant stressful life events, one or both of these emotional problems may occur (Barlow 2002).

In addition to this overlap, anxiety and depression also are very similar when you consider specific patterns of behaving. For example, as we mentioned earlier, eating and sleeping problems may be common to both conditions. Tendencies to abuse alcohol and other drugs also are related to both anxiety and depression. However, there is one exceptionally problematic behavioral tendency common to emotional disorders that, in our opinion, is the cornerstone for learning how to overcome these problems and have a more fulfilling quality of life. The focus of the next chapter, this behavioral pattern is called avoidance. *Avoidance* refers to the tendency to disengage from the world. It is about removing yourself or escaping from situations that elicit some fear or anxiety, or not engaging in behaviors that are difficult yet might bring about both short- and long-term rewards and pleasurable experiences. It's about being passive in our world, being fearful or unmotivated to behave in ways that would allow for a better life and more enjoyable experiences and social encounters. Avoidance is what causes your anxiety and depression to continue, and avoidance is what we must work toward changing.

CHAPTER 4

Understanding Avoidance in Your Life

TIME: Approximately One Week

There are many different ways to cope with difficult situations in your life. Some people prefer to confront problems very directly, working as quickly as they can to address certain issues and problems as soon as they develop. As a general example, if you have an argument with a coworker, you might choose to ask him or her to discuss the problem, work toward understanding what went wrong, and seek out a solution so that the problem doesn't happen again and there are no hard feelings. As an example specific to cancer, consider how you might cope with your diagnosis. For example, when you are diagnosed with cancer, one of the options is to do as much as possible to understand what cancer means, what the available treatment options are, what your prognosis is, and how you can live a lifestyle that may help to prevent reoccurrence of cancer once it is treated. Both examples involve what can be called *effective approach behavior.*

BEHAVIORAL AVOIDANCE

A very different strategy to cope with difficult situations involves the tendency to avoid. *Behavioral avoidance* is really about a reluctance or unwillingness to enter certain situations or get involved in certain behaviors or activities. So behavioral avoidance is evident in how you behave or, more accurately, your decision to not behave or engage in an action or activity. In other words, if a situation makes you uncomfortable or creates any anxiety or depressive feelings and you try to escape from that situation or simply do not put yourself it, you are behaviorally avoidant. This usually occurs as a result of believing that something bad will happen if you approach the situation or engage in a particular behavior. For example, if you noticed a lump in your breast or on your testicle, you might choose to try to ignore the situation and not seek medical consultation, possibly because you're afraid of what you might find out about the lump. Deciding not to show up for an appointment with your oncologist out of fear of what you might be told would be an example of behavioral avoidance. As another example, you may avoid certain social situations because you are depressed or anxious. The benefit of avoiding these situations is that you don't have to experience anxiety that may be created when you socialize. Because of a lack of pleasure you may have experienced in social situations in the past, you also may be more inclined to avoid socializing in the future and to be more passive, both of which might contribute to feeling more depressed.

Does Behavioral Avoidance Work?

It is very easy to avoid situations that are troublesome, cause you anxiety or fear, or have not provided you with positive experiences in the past. In fact, in several situations it is in your best interest to avoid. For example, if you come across an animal that seems to be acting aggressively, or have a spouse or partner who is verbally or physically abusive, or come across a drunken man who is shouting obscenities toward you, it is probably in your best interest to remove yourself from these situations so that you are unharmed and threats are removed.

EXERCISE: WHEN YOU SHOULD AVOID

Can you think of a few other situations in which it would make sense to avoid, or not become involved? If there are examples specific to your cancer, please be sure to list those here.

1. _____

2. _____

3. _____

In many situations, however, avoidance is not in your best interest. In the examples mentioned above, while avoidance may be useful in the short term to reduce anxiety, and you may be able to justify your avoidance based on previous experiences that were unpleasant, this avoidance also prevents you from overcoming your fear and learning that certain situations may actually be quite pleasurable. In other words, avoidance plays a major role in the continuation of your anxiety and depressive symptoms. The purpose of this chapter is to help you better understand situations and behaviors in your life that you may be avoiding and to link these avoidance tendencies to depression and anxiety symptoms.

EMOTIONAL AVOIDANCE

There are two general strategies that are used to avoid certain situations and experiences. Up to this stage, we have been talking about behavioral avoidance. Behavioral avoidance is a specific tendency that is part of a more general process of emotional avoidance.

What Is Emotional Avoidance?

Emotional avoidance refers to the tendency to be unwilling to remain in contact with (or to experience) certain sensations in your body, emotions, thoughts, memories, images, and desires to behave in particular ways (Hayes, Strosahl, and Wilson 1999). Because you do not want to have these experiences, you likely make some effort to avoid them. For example, you may be very uncomfortable when you begin to think about your cancer, what it means to be diagnosed with and live with cancer, how cancer has affected your life, and whether or not your life will be shortened because of cancer. As a result of this discomfort, you may attempt to suppress these thoughts and related emotions (such as sadness or anger), trying to push them out of your mind. On some level, this makes complete sense. After all, who wants to think about potentially painful things all the time, and who wants to experience some of the sadness or anger that may come with these thoughts?

Does Emotional Avoidance Work?

The problem is that we now have pretty good evidence to suggest that if you choose to cope with unwanted thoughts or feelings by trying to push them out of awareness, you may actually be increasing the likelihood of developing certain emotional problems like depression and anxiety (Barlow, Allen, and Choate 2004). For example, in an interesting study on war veterans, those individuals who were more unwilling to experience emotions (both positive and negative) were more likely to develop post-traumatic stress disorder (PTSD) than veterans willing to have emotional experiences (Roemer et al. 2001).

The message to be learned here is that with the exception of some genuinely threatening life events, behavioral avoidance does not help you to grow as an individual, and it also may cause you to develop and maintain problems with anxiety and depression. Second, the problem may not necessarily be that you actually have these negative thoughts, emotions, and memories, but rather that you try to force them away and avoid understanding and accepting them.

Consider this metaphor to better understand the problem of avoidance (Hayes, Strosahl, and Wilson 1999). You are walking alone in a jungle, enjoying the peacefulness of your surroundings, when all of a sudden you are approached by a little tiger. The tiger is small but is still somewhat frightening because he is an untamed animal. In your attempt to rid yourself of the tiger, you decide to give him a small piece of food that you're carrying in your backpack. To your great relief, the tiger takes the food and runs out of sight into the wilderness. However, we all know what happens when you feed an animal. They have learned where to find food and will likely want more. Sure enough, a short time later the tiger returns, and again, slightly more frightened this time, you provide the tiger with another piece of food. Thankfully, the tiger again grabs the food and retreats into the jungle. You walk along some more, and suddenly you are met by this same little tiger—and one that is substantially larger. Becoming more fearful, you again provide the tigers with food, they retreat, and this same pattern continues. More and more tigers become interested, and eventually (and most unfortunately) you run out of food. The lesson of this metaphor is that when you try to avoid certain situations and experiences, they can actually be made much worse. In this case, the alternative of experiencing and accepting the little tiger's visit might have more effectively resulted in his leaving. Instead, the act of trying to avoid him through providing food only complicated the matter.

So we hope that you will see that avoidance is in many circumstances a poor solution to dealing with problems. However, we also realize that, in the moment, it may feel like avoidance really is your best strategy. To help with this, a major theme of this workbook will be to help you to better understand your avoidance patterns, how they affect your life, and how to develop into a more active person who approaches situations—even those that are somewhat frightening or difficult to approach. Before we begin to explore the specific avoidance behaviors that you may engage in and how they affect you, let's take a look at how you may have become avoidant in the first place.

How People Become Avoidant

To begin looking at how avoidance develops, let's see how Jennifer began to experience it in relation to her health.

Jennifer awoke one Friday morning and did the typical things she had become used to doing. She showered and then took the dog out for a walk. When she returned, she gently awakened, dressed, and fed her little girl, began to drive her daughter to daycare, and thought about her plan for the day. She had gotten a few hours off of work so that she could attend her annual physical with her primary care physician. After the appointment she would grab a quick lunch and then head back to work.

As she sat in the doctor's waiting room, she thought about the paperwork that was sitting on her desk and the phone calls she had to make, hoping that she would be called back soon to meet with her doctor. Thankfully, she waited only fifteen minutes, and after being weighed and having her blood pressure taken, she was asked to wait for the doctor in one of the clinic rooms. A short time later, her doctor came in, asked her the usual questions, and then proceeded to conduct the physical examination. Jennifer continued to be preoccupied with thoughts of work and whether she would be able to get everything done before having to pick up her daughter. Then, seemingly out of nowhere, her doctor said, "Jennifer, how long have you had this lump on your left breast?" Jennifer was suddenly terrified. Her heart began to pound, she felt very dizzy, her thoughts started racing, and she felt like screaming. After feeling the rather large lump, she began to cry uncontrollably. "I haven't been doing my monthly self-exams," she said. "Do I have cancer?" "Well, let's not jump to any conclusions," replied her doctor. "It certainly is a suspicious lump, and I think we should schedule a biopsy. Even if it is cancer, Jennifer, please remember that the prognosis for breast cancer is very good, especially when it's detected early." A week later Jennifer found out that she did in fact have stage 1 breast cancer. She quickly received treatment, and after another evaluation several months later, was told that her cancer was in remission.

In several ways Jennifer's experience at the doctor's office was a good one. She learned of a medical problem she had, received support from her physician, and followed up with a very successful treatment that involved surgery and radiation therapy. However, Jennifer also associated the doctor's visit with anxiety and fear, emotions she experienced when being told she might have cancer. In large part due to this experience, and despite the positive aspects of attending her appointment on that day, Jennifer decided that physician's offices caused her a lot of discomfort. As a result of this discomfort, Jennifer still has not been back to see her primary care physician or oncologist, even a year and a half after the end of her treatment.

Situations like this happen all the time in our world. Not all of us necessarily get diagnosed with cancer, but all of us do find ourselves in situations that are uncomfortable or cause certain degrees of fear, anxiety, anger, sadness, or guilt. Because few of us enjoy experiencing these kinds of emotions, we often choose to limit our experiences with them. This means that we avoid situations that might cause these emotional reactions and also often avoid thinking about these situations. Unfortunately, these tendencies to avoid can have serious consequences. In Jennifer's case, it's clear what the consequences of avoiding doctors might be. Without further medical observation, there is a chance her cancer could return and remain undetected, potentially becoming a more serious (or metastatic) form of cancer. She also may have other medical problems that would remain undetected and untreated.

AVOIDANCE IS LEARNED

The point to be made here is that avoidance behavior is learned. We learn to avoid certain situations, events, experiences, or people because they have been associated in some way with a negative experience. Sometimes we learn to avoid because of direct learning experiences, as Jennifer did. Other times we learn to avoid through observing others having negative experiences, or simply through being told about or receiving information about negative experiences. For example, Jennifer could have developed her avoidance of doctor's offices if she had accompanied a friend to an appointment in which her friend was diagnosed with breast cancer and had a negative emotional reaction. She also could have developed an avoidance pattern as the result of reading an article about breast cancer and chemotherapy that focused on the potential side effects of chemotherapy.

AVOIDANCE CAN BE UNLEARNED

The good news is that just as avoidance behaviors can be learned, they can also be unlearned. Why is it essential to learn how to more effectively approach situations? Well, for one thing, if you are avoidant or passive, these tendencies may prevent you from recognizing or solving problems in your life, problems that may contribute to feeling depressed and anxious. Jennifer's situation illustrates this issue. Her avoidance may prevent her from recognizing medical problems, and although she may feel less anxious or depressed in the short term by avoiding, you might imagine how finding out about a return of her cancer (in possibly a more severe form) at a later time would make her feel even worse. As other examples, think about how avoiding a social interaction with a romantic partner, a problem that you have with your coworkers in the workplace, or getting exercise at a local recreation center might serve to maintain problems in your life, problems that may have a major impact on your emotional state.

IS AVOIDANCE A PROBLEM FOR YOU?

Given the problem with avoidance and its strong relationship to feelings of depression and anxiety, we now turn our focus toward helping you better understand the extent to which avoidance is a problem in your life. To accomplish this goal, we ask you to answer some questions about a number of different life areas in which avoidance may be a central problem. In chapter 5, we'll teach you how to overcome your avoidance, anxiety, and depression by learning to behave differently using behavioral activation.

EXERCISE: MEASURING THE EXTENT OF YOUR AVOIDANCE

In the space provided below, and paying attention to the specific questions presented, indicate whether you feel avoidance is evident in these areas of your life.

1. **Family relationships.** Within your family system (for instance, parents, children, uncles, aunts, cousins, grandparents, *but not spouse or partner*), think about those relationships in which you feel somewhat unhappy, dissatisfied, or unfulfilled. Write down the names of these individuals.

    _____

    _____

    _____

    Now, write down what you think the primary problems are in these relationships, focusing on what you may be saying or doing that may be contributing to the problem, as well as what the other person may be saying or doing to contribute to the problem.

    _____

    _____

    _____

    Now, ask yourself what you might say or do differently to try to resolve the problem. Focus on yourself. It is difficult to try to change or control the actions of others. What might you do to try to make the situation better?

    _____

    _____

    _____

    Have you tried to do these things? YES/NO (Circle one). If yes, why hasn't it worked? Are there different strategies you might try? If no, why haven't you tried? Why are you avoiding the opportunity to try to make things better? Are you fearful of something? What obstacles stand in your way?

    _____

    _____

Is avoiding the situation helping you or making the situation (including your anxiety or depression) worse?

_____

_____

What plan can you come up with for overcoming your fear or concerns about the situation? How can you overcome the obstacles? How can you approach the situation?

_____

_____

_____

2. **Social relationships.** Think about those friendships or acquaintance relationships in which you feel somewhat unhappy, dissatisfied, or unfulfilled. Write down the names of these people.

_____

_____

_____

Now, write down what you think the primary problems are in these relationships, focusing on what you may be saying or doing that may be contributing to the problem, as well as what the other person may be saying or doing to contribute to the problem.

_____

_____

_____

Now, ask yourself what you might say or do differently to try to resolve the problem. Again, focus on yourself. It is difficult to try to change or control the actions of others. What might you do to try to make the situation better?

_____

_____

_____

Have you tried to do these things? YES/NO (Circle one). If yes, why hasn't it worked? Are there different strategies you might try? If no, why haven't you tried? Why are you avoiding the opportunity to try to make things better? Are you fearful of something? What obstacles stand in your way?

_____

_____

_____

Is avoiding the situation helping you or making the situation (including your anxiety or depression) worse?

_____

_____

What plan can you come up with for overcoming your fear or concerns about the situation? How can you overcome the obstacles? How can you approach the situation?

_____

_____

_____

3.   **Intimate relationships.** Think about aspects of the relationship you have with your spouse or partner that make you feel somewhat unhappy, dissatisfied, or unfulfilled. Now, write down what you think the primary problems are in this relationship, focusing on what you may be saying or doing that may be contributing to the problem, as well as what the other person may be saying or doing to contribute.

_____

_____

_____

Now, ask yourself what you might say or do differently to try to resolve the problem. Focus on yourself. What might you do to try to make the situation better?

_____

_____

_____

Have you tried to do these things? YES/NO (Circle one). If yes, why hasn't it worked? Are there different strategies you might try? If no, why haven't you tried? Why are you avoiding the opportunity to try to make things better? Are you fearful of something? What obstacles stand in your way?

_____

_____

_____

Is avoiding the situation helping you or making the situation (including your anxiety or depression) worse?

_____

_____

What plan can you come up with for overcoming your fear or concerns about the situation? How can you overcome the obstacles? How can you approach the situation?

_____

_____

_____

4. **Limited relationships.** In doing the preceding three sections, did it become clear to you that you have a limited social support system (recall the exercise in chapter 1 on social support)? Write down what you think the primary problems might be that stand in the way of developing a better social system, focusing on what you may be saying or doing that may be contributing to the problem, as well as what other people may be saying or doing to contribute to the problem.

_____

_____

_____

Now, ask yourself what you might say or do differently to try to resolve the problem. Focus on yourself. What might you do to provide more opportunities to increase your social network?

_____

_____

_____

Have you tried to do these things? YES/NO (Circle one). If yes, why hasn't it worked? Are there different strategies you might try? If no, why haven't you tried? Why are you avoiding the opportunity to try to increase your social network? Are you fearful of something? What obstacles stand in your way?

_____

_____

_____

Is avoiding social situations helping you or making your life (including your anxiety or depression) worse?

_____

_____

What plan can you come up with for overcoming your fear or concerns about the situation? How can you overcome the obstacles? How can you approach social situations?

_____

_____

_____

5. **Education/training.** Think about how you feel about your education, level of intelligence, and training experiences. Do you feel happy, satisfied, and fulfilled?

_____

_____

_____

Are there ways to become more satisfied or fulfilled with this aspect of your life? Are there intellectual activities or educational experiences that you would like to pursue? If yes, what are these experiences? Be as specific as possible.

_____

_____

_____

Now, write down why you think you haven't pursued these opportunities. Why are you avoiding the opportunity to improve this aspect of your life? Are you fearful of something? What obstacles stand in your way?

_____

_____

_____

Is avoiding the situation helping you or making the situation (including your anxiety or depression) worse?

_____

_____

What might you do to try to resolve this problem and make the situation better? What plan can you come up with for overcoming your fear or concerns about the situation, and how can you overcome the obstacles so you can approach the situation?

_____

_____

_____

6. **Employment/career.** Think about your current employment situation and your career choice. Do you feel happy, satisfied, and fulfilled?

_____

_____

_____

Are there ways to become more satisfied or fulfilled with this aspect of your life? Are there employment or career opportunities that you would like to pursue? If yes, what are these experiences? Be as specific as possible.

_____

_____

_____

Now, write down why you think you haven't pursued these opportunities. Why are you avoiding the opportunity to improve this aspect of your life? Are you fearful of something? What obstacles stand in your way?

_____

_____

_____

Is avoiding the situation helping you or making the situation (including your anxiety or depression) worse?

_____

_____

What might you do to try to resolve this problem and make the situation better? What plan can you come up with for overcoming your fear or concerns about the situation, and how can you overcome the obstacles so you can approach the situation?

_____

_____

_____

7. **Hobbies/recreation.** Think about how you feel about the hobbies or recreational experiences that are part of your life. Do you feel happy, satisfied, and fulfilled?

_____

_____

_____

Are there ways to become more satisfied or fulfilled with this aspect of your life? Is there something missing? Are there hobbies or recreational activities that you would like to pursue? If yes, what are these experiences? Be as specific as possible.

_____

_____

_____

Now, write down why you think you haven't pursued these opportunities. Why are you avoiding the opportunity to improve this aspect of your life? Are you fearful of something? What obstacles stand in your way?

_____

_____

_____

Is avoiding the situation helping you, or is it perhaps reducing your satisfaction with life (including increasing anxiety or depression)?

_____

_____

What might you do to try to resolve this problem and make the situation better? What plan can you come up with for overcoming your fear or concerns about the situation, and how can you overcome the obstacles so you can approach the situation?

_____

_____

_____

8. **Volunteer work/charity/political activities.** Think about how you feel about the volunteer work, charities, and political groups that you may belong to. Do you feel happy, satisfied, and fulfilled?

_____

_____

_____

Are there ways to become more satisfied or fulfilled with this aspect of your life? If yes, what are these experiences? Be as specific as possible.

_____

_____

_____

Now, write down why you think you haven't pursued these opportunities. Why are you avoiding the opportunity to improve this aspect of your life? Are you fearful of something? What obstacles stand in your way?

_____

_____

_____

Is avoiding the situation helping you or making your life (including your anxiety or depression) worse?

_____

_____

What might you do to try to resolve this problem and make the situation better? What plan can you come up with for overcoming your fear or concerns about the situation, and how can you overcome the obstacles so you can approach the situation?

_____

_____

_____

9. **Physical/health issues.** Think about how you feel about your physical health. Do you feel happy, satisfied, and fulfilled?

_____

_____

_____

Are there ways to become more satisfied or fulfilled with your physical health and fitness? Are there health-related experiences that you would like to pursue? If yes, what are these experiences? Be as specific as possible.

_____

_____

_____

Now, write down why you think you haven't pursued these opportunities. Why are you avoiding the opportunity to improve this aspect of your life? Are you fearful of something? What obstacles stand in your way?

_____

_____

_____

Is avoiding the situation helping you or making your life less rewarding (including increasing anxiety or depression)?

_____

_____

What might you do to try to resolve this problem and make the situation better? What plan can you come up with for overcoming your fear or concerns about the situation, and how can you overcome the obstacles so you can approach the situation?

_____

_____

_____

10. **Spirituality.** Think about how you feel about your spirituality or religious affiliations. Do you feel happy, satisfied, and fulfilled?

_____

_____

_____

Are there ways to become more satisfied or fulfilled in your spiritual life? Are there religious or spiritual activities that you would like to pursue? If yes, what are these experiences? Be as specific as possible.

_____

_____

_____

Now, write down why you think you haven't pursued these opportunities. Why are you avoiding the opportunity to improve this aspect of your life? Are you fearful of something? What obstacles stand in your way?

_____

_____

_____

Is avoiding the situation helping you or making your life less satisfying (including maybe increasing your anxiety and depression)?

_____

_____

What might you do to try to resolve this problem and make the situation better? What plan can you come up with for overcoming your fear or concerns about the situation, and how can you overcome the obstacles so you can approach the situation?

_____

_____

_____

11. **Situations that cause you to feel fearful, anxious, or depressed.** Think about situations that cause you to feel fearful, anxious, or depressed. Please think about this carefully, and specifically indicate what these situations are (for instance, where you are, who is there, what is going on).

_____

_____

_____

To what extent do you avoid these situations? What are you fearful of? What obstacles stand in the way of approaching these situations?

_____

_____

Keeping in mind our earlier discussion of emotional avoidance—the tendency to be unwilling to remain in contact with (or experience) certain sensations in your body, emotions, thoughts, memories, or images—are there certain things you try to do when you feel an uncomfortable emotion such as depression or anxiety? Do you engage in some task, distract yourself, procrastinate, zone out in front of the television? What do you do when you feel an uncomfortable emotion?

_____

_____

_____

Is avoiding situations, thoughts, or emotional experiences helping you, or is it perhaps making your life less rewarding?

_____

_____

What might you do to try to resolve this problem and make the situation better? What plan can you come up with for overcoming your fear or concerns about the situation, and how can you overcome the obstacles so you can approach the situation?

_____

_____

_____

Now that we have clearly highlighted your patterns of avoidance in a number of very important life areas, we have a much clearer picture of the behaviors we need to focus on in the behavioral activation component of this workbook. Although additional coping strategies will be presented later on, this is the primary strategy we will use to teach you to take charge of your life, eliminate avoidance behaviors and become more active in your world, experience a more rewarding lifestyle, and subsequently overcome your feelings of depression and anxiety.

CHAPTER 5

Behavioral Activation Treatment for Cancer (BAT-C)

During the next ten weeks, you will be participating in a treatment referred to as *behavioral activation*. As you may recall from chapter 2, behavioral activation was designed to help you increase the frequency of healthy behaviors and the pleasure that you experience from engaging in these behaviors. This process involves assisting you to learn new ways of behaving and helping you to reduce kinds of avoidance (that you outlined in the previous chapter) that may serve to maintain your depression and anxiety.

As you will notice, this is a lengthier chapter that presents the major intervention in this book. As such, it may appear somewhat overwhelming at first glance. However, we assure you that although a lot of information is presented here, we have arranged the chapter so that you will not feel overwhelmed and will be able to move at a pace that is comfortable to you. You have already made tremendous strides toward learning more about your cancer and how it is related to your depression, anxiety, and avoidance behavior. Now comes the exciting part—learning how to better cope with these emotions and developing a lifestyle that will allow you to feel more fulfilled in your life.

WEEK 1: GETTING STARTED

To begin your process of learning to activate, we will provide you with a brief history of how behavioral activation came to be developed. Secondly, getting you on the path of learning how to more effectively spend your time and experience increased pleasure and reward in your life, we will guide you through the initial step of better understanding how you currently spend your time and help you identify where some problems might exist.

Although some of the strategies and theories that characterize behavioral activation have been around for about thirty years, the behavioral activation treatment in its current form has been around for about a decade (Jacobson et al. 1996). Following from this initial study that indicated behavioral activation might be a useful approach to reduce depression, treatment manuals were developed to assist people in overcoming symptoms of depression (Addis and Martell 2004; Lejuez, Hopko, and Hopko 2002; Martell, Addis, and Jacobson 2001). Over the past five years, these approaches have been effectively used to treat people with depression and anxiety, and perhaps most importantly for you, people who have cancer and are also depressed and anxious (Dimidjian et al. 2006; Hopko et al. 2005, 2006). Importantly, there also is some good evidence to suggest behavioral activation may be as effective as medication in reducing depressive symptoms and may even result in longer-term treatment gains and reduced medical costs (Dimidjian et al. 2006). Considering these very positive findings, there is every reason to believe that behavioral activation might be a useful intervention to assist you in overcoming your feelings of depression and anxiety.

How Behavioral Activation Treatment Works

The treatment that we will be teaching you is based on the belief that the best way to reduce depression and anxiety symptoms and to make long-term changes in your life is by looking at how you spend your time, understanding what is important in your life (your values), and then changing the nature of the activities in which you currently are engaged to make your behaviors more consistent with your values and goals in life. In other words, we are going to teach you a different way of behaving that will make it more likely that you will experience more positive and enjoyable situations. It's much more difficult to feel depressed or anxious and have low self-esteem if you are regularly engaging in activities that bring you a sense of pleasure and/or accomplishment.

Keep in mind that it is possible to be quite active yet still depressed or anxious. This might happen when activities occur often but are not very fulfilling or gratifying to you. In other words, the activities may be inconsistent with your life goals and values. For example, although you may be active at work, earn a good income, and complete chores at home, sacrificing time and activities with your child or spouse (an important life goal) may result in depressive emotions. Thus, it's not how often you engage in different activities but rather how rewarding or gratifying these activities are for you.

This treatment is behavioral in nature, which means that we will work toward changing your behavior (how you spend your time) as a method for improving your thoughts, mood, and overall quality of life. People with depression and anxiety often feel very passive and lack the motivation to engage in various activities. Depressed people often think that once they have more energy and think more positively, they will be able to engage in activities they have ignored or have been unable to accomplish.

The very opposite approach is taken in this treatment. Here, behavior is changed first, despite feelings of depression or anxiety that you may be experiencing. In other words, we ask you to think about changing the way you spend your time despite how you may feel. This may sound tough at first, but we assure you that it is very possible for you to do if you commit to the idea. In fact, we all do this in various situations. For example, many people wake up in the morning and do not feel like going to work. There are a hundred other things they would rather be doing. However, because of the rewards that come from going to work—including financial gain, experiences of achievement, and maybe rewarding social interactions—more often than not, people go to work despite a desire to do something else. As another example, when you were being treated for your cancer, maybe through radiation therapy or chemotherapy, there probably were many other ways you would rather have spent your time. However, because of the desire to treat the cancer and get well, you chose to undergo treatment despite your wishes and desires to spend your time in more enjoyable ways.

So you can see that it's possible to behave in a way that is somewhat inconsistent with the way you feel. That is a good thing, because it allows you to try to change your feelings and emotions by behaving differently. Once you change certain behaviors, we believe you will then see fairly dramatic changes in your energy level, motivation, positive thinking, and moods (less depressed and anxious). Please remember that in focusing on behavior change, we do not ignore thoughts and feelings. Instead, we suggest that negative thoughts and feelings will change only after you change your behavior and are experiencing positive events and consequences more frequently.

To put this in a slightly different way, we basically take an acceptance-versus-change approach to treatment. Some things in your life are very difficult to control or change. These things might include what other people say or do (it's hard to control people), particular thoughts that we have (it's often difficult to stop thinking about certain things), or certain life experiences that we have (for example, being diagnosed with cancer). These are things that you can't do much about changing. Thus, your only alternative is to work more toward accepting that there are things you can't change, such as being diagnosed and treated for cancer. On the other hand, there are situations that you do have the ability to change if you take the steps necessary to accomplish these changes. If it helps to put this in a different perspective, and particularly if you are a spiritual person, think about the serenity prayer: God, grant me the serenity to accept the things I cannot change, courage to change the things I can, and the wisdom to know the difference between the two. Consistent with the philosophy behind the serenity prayer, there is one thing that you really do have the power to change. Specifically, that's how you behave, the activities that you do, and the way you spend your time. So that's what we're going to focus on in this treatment.

To make it easier to work toward changing behavior, it's often useful to think about behavior as either "depressed or anxious" or "healthy" behavior. Actions related to your depression and anxiety symptoms are your depressed or anxious behaviors. For example, these behaviors might include being avoidant (as we have already spoken about), being passive or inactive, watching a lot of television, and sleeping excessively. On the other hand, we refer to positive actions that are inconsistent with depressed and anxious behaviors as *healthy behavior*. Healthy behavior is directed toward improving your life and is generally focused on attaining some goal, objective, or reward. The goal of this treatment is to assist you in learning how to behave in a healthier way in a number of different life areas. These life areas, which we addressed in chapter 4, include such things as relationships, recreational activities and hobbies, exercise, spirituality, work, education, leisure activities, learning activities, and household activities. Rest assured that we are aware that you may have physical limitations because of current cancer symptoms or involvement in treatment. However, we believe that even under these conditions, there are possible steps you can take to change your behavior and improve your emotional well-being.

Why This Treatment Can Be Useful for You

There are several reasons why the behavioral activation treatment for cancer (BAT-C) may be very useful for you. First, as we mentioned above, preliminary outcome studies of behavioral activation strategies with cancer patients are highly encouraging. Second, many of the other psychological treatment options that are available to you are quite complicated and would take extensive training and skill to be able to do yourself. Third, many of these other available treatments require a significant time commitment, some lasting for several years. The strategies we offer in this workbook are much more time-efficient. Importantly, if you are in the midst of ongoing cancer treatment (or just recovering from treatment) that may be time consuming and physically and emotionally overwhelming, additional time demands of behavioral activation are minimal. Fourth, because behavioral activation treatment encourages healthy, nondepressed behavior, and considering limitations in behaviors and increased problems and daily hassles reported by cancer patients (Ciaramella and Poli 2001; Nezu et al. 1999), this intervention may be optimal in helping you with behavior change and improving your mood. Fifth, BAT-C also involves increasing a sense of control over your life (and your behavior), a characteristic that may be useful in combating the loss of control often experienced by cancer patients. Behavioral activation also addresses important aspects of cancer treatment that include social and family support, emotional expression, reordering of life priorities, and symptom control. Sixth, BAT-C does not have the side effects that may be associated with antidepressant or antianxiety medications, a fact that may be particularly desirable for cancer patients who are already undergoing chemotherapy or radiotherapy. Seventh, given the vast differences among cancer patients in terms of their backgrounds, values in life, treatment goals, and psychological and medical symptoms, the flexible nature of behavioral activation allows treatment to be tailored to your unique needs. Finally, it is known that medical patients receiving behavior therapy may experience less pain, decreased medication usage, and less frequent medical visits (Hopko et al. 2005, 2006). Therefore, cancer patients who receive BAT-C may experience not only reduced depressive and anxiety symptoms but also more coping resources, fewer medical problems, fewer visits to your physicians, and perhaps fewer antidepressant and antianxiety medications.

Preparing to Begin Behavioral Activation Treatment

To begin any treatment, you must be motivated to make a commitment to do your best to follow the recommendations that are given to you. Whether or not this treatment is effective for you will in large part be determined by how much effort you put into following the suggestions given to you. We would like you to think about participating in this treatment in the same way you would think about receiving a medical treatment. For example, if you had a throat infection and were prescribed an antibiotic, your doctor would inform you to make sure to take the entire prescription, at certain times, and until you had taken all of the pills, even if you were already feeling better part of the way through treatment. Only then would you be assured that the bacteria had been completely destroyed.

The same logic applies to this treatment, only it is a different kind of prescription. It doesn't involve you having to take medication at a certain time each day, but it involves requiring you to complete practice exercises and engage in different behaviors at scheduled times. Only if you follow this prescription of behavior can you expect to achieve the maximum benefit, just like taking the antibiotics. Of course, we understand that it might be easier to commit yourself to taking a couple of pills a day for one week than to commit yourself to learning how to behave differently over the course of ten weeks. For this reason, we need to clearly emphasize why it's important that you make this commitment, as well as highlight some of the barriers that may stand in the way of your completing treatment, so that if certain obstacles come up, they can be addressed to make it easier for you to follow the treatment guidelines.

DO YOU NEED TO CHANGE?

As we mentioned in the introduction, this workbook is appropriate for people with cancer who are feeling depressed or anxious or who are fearful or saddened by having to live with cancer. If you have these emotional experiences, odds are that this book will be useful toward helping you lead a more fulfilling life that is not clouded by these negative emotions. Moving beyond experiencing symptoms of depression and anxiety, this workbook will be particularly helpful if you are having significant problems with living. In other words, sometimes feelings of depression and anxiety can be so strong that people are unable to follow through with their regular daily routines. For example, depression and anxiety can be so problematic that you may be unable to work, cook, or take care of your children. You could also find that you may be isolating yourself from others so that you have reduced social support from friends and family, are having marital or relationship problems, have decreased job satisfaction or unemployment, or are not succeeding in pursuing your educational goals or other opportunities for intellectual growth. You also may have given up on previously rewarding or pleasurable hobbies and activities.

In addition, there may be psychological consequences to your depression and anxiety that may include decreased optimism and motivation,. low self-esteem, feelings of hopelessness or helplessness, difficulty concentrating, and possibly extreme reactions such as the desire to hurt yourself and even possibly think about suicide. Finally, there may be medical consequences of depression and anxiety that could include a worsening of physical conditions such as cancer or heart disease and maybe even an increased tendency to abuse alcohol or other drugs, increased fatigue, decreased appetite, and even malnutrition.

EXERCISE: REASONS TO MAKE SOME CHANGES IN YOUR LIFE

Take a moment to think about these issues and write down why you think it's time for a change in your life. How has depression and anxiety affected you, and why is it time to do things differently?

_____

_____

_____

_____

Sometimes, even though people recognize that depression or anxiety is having a negative impact on their life, they feel like they are in such a deep hole that it's impossible for them to climb out. We understand that change is difficult, and it is normal to have mixed emotions about the process of changing your behavior. For example, if you are depressed, you may think "I'm so unhappy with my life, and I wish that I could just do more things that would make me happy, like spending time with people, exercising more, and engaging in all the activities that used to bring a smile to my face." At the same time, however, you may also be thinking, "But I don't feel like I have a lot to offer to other people. I feel like a burden, I have no self-esteem, and change just seems too hard." If you are anxious, you may want to face the experiences and situations that make you anxious or fearful. At the same time, these situations may be so frightening that the mere thought of putting yourself in those situations makes you feel terrified and even paralyzed, and you quickly think of something else so you don't have to even consider facing your fears. Going back and forth with these thoughts is a normal human experience.

To help you to further evaluate your readiness to change, many people find it helpful to think about their present self as compared to their ideal self. Your _present self_ refers to how you currently view your life. Your _ideal self_ refers to the person you want to be, in an ideal world. The ideal you is the way you want to define yourself and the way you hope others will see you and remember you.

EXERCISE: WHO YOU ARE AND WHO YOU WANT TO BECOME

Take a couple of minutes to think about your life, your family, your relationships, your health and fitness, your work or educational experiences, your hobbies and recreational activities, and your spirituality. Are you where you want to be? How big is the discrepancy between your present self and ideal self? Is there a lot of room for improvement in various aspects of your life? What areas of your life are in need of the most change?

_____

_____

_____

_____

_____

_____

_____

_____

_____

In finishing this exercise, remember that the more progress you can make in closing the gap between your present self and your ideal self, the more you will feel fulfilled and the less you will feel depressed and anxious. This is precisely the objective of behavioral activation therapy, providing a strategy that will help you reduce the avoidance in your life and allow you to behave differently so that you can more closely resemble your ideal self and experience the positive emotions that come with making this change.

DEPRESSION AND ANXIETY

So, one reason why it's important for you to make changes in your life is to make the transition from your present self to your ideal self. Another obvious reason is that you are probably uncomfortable with the feelings of depression and anxiety you have come to experience. When you think about your feeling of depression and anxiety and the impact these emotions have had on your life, using the scale below, how important would you say it is for you to become less depressed and anxious?

0	1	2	3	4	5	6	7	8	9	10
Not at all important										Extremely important

Now, how confident are you that if you decided to work toward becoming less depressed and anxious, you could do it?

0	1	2	3	4	5	6	7	8	9	10
Not at all confident										Extremely confident

For the moment, it is more critical that you feel as though it is important to change your feelings of depression and anxiety. Although it is wonderful if you feel a high level of confidence in your ability to do so, it is understandable if you don't feel terribly confident. A lack of confidence may be due to many circumstances, including but not limited to unsuccessful previous attempts to decrease depression and anxiety; current feelings of fatigue and weakness that may be related to depression, anxiety, and cancer symptoms and treatment; or ongoing life stressors you believe might stand in the way of making progress. For now, know that we are aware that you may not feel 100 percent confident—and that's okay. We will work at a pace that helps you to build your confidence and ensure that you get as much as possible out of treatment.

Try to remember that there are both pros and cons associated with making the commitment to change.

PROS of change:

Fewer depressive thoughts and feelings

Fewer problems with stress and anxiety

Health benefits from decreased depression/stress

Research suggests better mental health may reduce physical problems

Cancer symptoms may become less problematic and easier to live with

Function better—more energy

CONS of change:

Takes time/energy to read this workbook

Takes time/energy to practice exercises

EXERCISE: ADDRESSING YOUR POTENTIAL OBSTACLES TO CHANGE

When you think about these pros and cons and your current life circumstances, what do you think would be some potential obstacles to your making changes and engaging in treatment? These obstacles might include a busy work schedule, limited time to read this workbook and engage in practice exercises, limited social support to help you through this process, cancer-related pain and fatigue, and so forth. What potential solutions can you come up with to resolve these issues?

_____

_____

_____

_____

_____

_____

_____

_____

Monitoring Already Occurring Daily Activities

Because the main focus of this treatment is increasing your level of healthy behavior and decreasing avoidance behavior, it is important to get an accurate assessment of your current daily activities. The reality is that you are currently feeling depressed and/or anxious, and these emotions are in all probability related to how you're spending your time. Although you may believe that you have a good idea of how you spend each day, most people have certain behaviors and routines that have become so automatic that they may not even be aware of how often they occur or how they may be affecting mood. There may be certain patterns of behaving that may be unrewarding in your life and might be contributing to your feeling depressed or anxious.

To illustrate how this may occur, consider the situation of Robert. Robert was a successful architect who earned a nice salary and had a comfortable home in the suburbs of a large city. He was happily married and had two young children, ages two and six. Robert was diagnosed with prostate cancer approximately a year ago, but it had been treated and there were no signs of recurrence. In fact, Robert indicated that he had experienced little in the way of major life stressors in the past six months. Yet he found himself to be profoundly depressed. His mood was down, he was not engaging in previously enjoyable activities (going to church, going on hikes in the woods, playing video games), and he was feeling tremendously guilty and had low self-esteem. Robert's therapist asked him to complete a daily diary exercise where he would record how he was spending his time. This record would help determine if there were noticeable patterns that might be contributing to his depression. As part of this exercise, Robert recorded not only how he was spending his time but also how much pleasure he was experiencing when engaged in various activities. One of his daily diaries (Sunday) is presented here.

M T W TH F SA(SU)		Pleasurable? 1 (least) – 4 (most)
8:00–8:30 A.M.	Had breakfast	3
8:30–9:00 A.M.	Showered	3
9:00–9:30 A.M.	Drove to work	2
9:30–10:00 A.M.	Worked on new contract	2
10:00–10:30 A.M.		2
10:30–11:00 A.M.		2
11:00–11:30 A.M.		2
11:30 A.M.–12:00 P.M.		2
12:00–12:30 P.M.	Had lunch	3
12:30–1:00 P.M.	Continued to work on new contract	1
1:00–1:30 P.M.		1
1:30–2:00 P.M.		1
2:00–2:30 P.M.		1
2:30–3:00 P.M.		1
3:00–3:30 P.M.		1
3:30–4:00 P.M.		1
4:00–4:30 P.M.		1
4:30–5:00 P.M.		1
5:00–5:30 P.M.	Drove home from work	2
5:30–6:00 P.M.	Had dinner with wife and kids	3
6:00–6:30 P.M.		3
6:30–7:00 P.M.	Read bedtime story to children	4
7:00–7:30 P.M.	Cleaned garage	2
7:30–8:00 P.M.	Watched movie with my wife	3
8:00–8:30 P.M.		3
8:30–9:00 P.M.		3
9:00–9:30 P.M.		3
9:30–10:00 P.M.	Went to sleep	3
10:00–10:30 P.M.		3
10:30–11:00 P.M.		3
11:00–11:30 P.M.		3
11:30 P.M.–12:00 A.M.		3

When Robert and his therapist reviewed his daily monitoring exercise, they made a few very important observations. First, Robert had not engaged in activities that used to bring him a great deal of satisfaction. Second, because of an increasing number of contracts that Robert was responsible for, he was spending a considerable amount of time working on the weekends. Although he almost always gave high pleasure ratings to his work during the week, Robert found work much less satisfying on the weekend. Third, because of his weekend work schedule, Robert was neglecting (or avoiding) other important aspects of his life, particularly being involved with his children. After further discussion with his therapist, Robert had an interesting realization about how his behavior was related to his mood. He realized that his increased work commitments had triggered his depressive feelings in that he was spending more time in the office and not going to church, hiking, or playing video games. But more importantly, he realized that it was not the activities themselves that brought him a sense of pleasure (he actually did hike once during the week but found it unrewarding). Rather, it was the fact that prior to his work commitments increasing, going to church, hiking, and playing video games were activities he did with his children. The absence of these activities was greatly decreasing his life satisfaction, was inconsistent with his value system, and was strongly related to his depression. Without completing the daily monitoring exercise, Robert and his therapist might not have realized this set of circumstances.

Just as Robert and his therapist learned a great deal from reviewing his daily diary exercise, you may learn a lot about the way you are spending your time, how rewarding certain activities are, what behavioral patterns might be evident, and how your behaviors might be related to your feelings of depression and anxiety. So for the next seven days, we would like you to monitor your current activities. This may be useful for several reasons. First, it provides an initial measurement to evaluate your progress when you have increased your activity level later in treatment. Second, looking at your current level of activity may enable you to realize that you have certain behavioral patterns, are maybe less active than you originally thought, or are spending large amounts of time engaging in unhealthy, depressed behavior. Seeing evidence of this may provide motivation for you to increase your healthy activity level. Finally, a close examination of your daily routine might help you to develop some ideas as to what behaviors and activities might make you feel more fulfilled.

EXERCISE: HOW DO YOU SPEND YOUR TIME?

For the next seven days, please keep a detailed record of your activities, including those that seem insignificant, such as sleeping or watching television. As much as possible during this week, just do what you typically do. Write down your behaviors during half-hour intervals. You don't have to put everything you did in each half hour, only how you spent most of your time during that half hour. Only record your behaviors—what you do and how you spend your time. Don't write down specific thoughts or feelings you might be having. Also, don't worry about writing down everything as it happens. Instead, try to keep track of your behaviors every three to four hours, remembering how you spent your time. When you write down your behaviors, rate each of them using the scale provided, from 1 (least pleasurable) to 4 (most pleasurable). You have one form for each day of the week. Try to be as accurate and as thorough as you can.

M T W TH F SA SU		Pleasurable? 1 (least) – 4 (most)
6:00–6:30 A.M.		
6:30–7:00 A.M.		
7:00–7:30 A.M.		
7:30–8:00 A.M.		
8:00–8:30 A.M.		
8:30–9:00 A.M.		
9:00–9:30 A.M.		
9:30–10:00 A.M.		
10:00–10:30 A.M.		
10:30–11:00 A.M.		
11:00–11:30 A.M.		
11:30 A.M.–12:00 P.M.		
12:00–12:30 P.M.		
12:30–1:00 P.M.		
1:00–1:30 P.M.		
1:30–2:00 P.M.		
2:00–2:30 P.M.		
2:30–3:00 P.M.		
3:00–3:30 P.M.		
3:30–4:00 P.M.		
4:00–4:30 P.M.		
4:30–5:00 P.M.		
5:00–5:30 P.M.		
5:30–6:00 P.M.		
6:00–6:30 P.M.		
6:30–7:00 P.M.		
7:00–7:30 P.M.		
7:30–8:00 P.M.		
8:00–8:30 P.M.		
8:30–9:00 P.M.		
9:00–9:30 P.M.		
9:30–10:00 P.M.		
10:00–10:30 P.M.		
10:30–11:00 P.M.		
11:00–11:30 P.M.		
11:30 P.M.–12:00 A.M.		

M T W TH F SA SU		Pleasurable? 1 (least) – 4 (most)
6:00–6:30 A.M.		
6:30–7:00 A.M.		
7:00–7:30 A.M.		
7:30–8:00 A.M.		
8:00–8:30 A.M.		
8:30–9:00 A.M.		
9:00–9:30 A.M.		
9:30–10:00 A.M.		
10:00–10:30 A.M.		
10:30–11:00 A.M.		
11:00–11:30 A.M.		
11:30 A.M.–12:00 P.M.		
12:00–12:30 P.M.		
12:30–1:00 P.M.		
1:00–1:30 P.M.		
1:30–2:00 P.M.		
2:00–2:30 P.M.		
2:30–3:00 P.M.		
3:00–3:30 P.M.		
3:30–4:00 P.M.		
4:00–4:30 P.M.		
4:30–5:00 P.M.		
5:00–5:30 P.M.		
5:30–6:00 P.M.		
6:00–6:30 P.M.		
6:30–7:00 P.M.		
7:00–7:30 P.M.		
7:30–8:00 P.M.		
8:00–8:30 P.M.		
8:30–9:00 P.M.		
9:00–9:30 P.M.		
9:30–10:00 P.M.		
10:00–10:30 P.M.		
10:30–11:00 P.M.		
11:00–11:30 P.M.		
11:30 P.M.–12:00 A.M.		

M T W TH F SA SU		Pleasurable? 1 (least) – 4 (most)
6:00–6:30 A.M.		
6:30–7:00 A.M.		
7:00–7:30 A.M.		
7:30–8:00 A.M.		
8:00–8:30 A.M.		
8:30–9:00 A.M.		
9:00–9:30 A.M.		
9:30–10:00 A.M.		
10:00–10:30 A.M.		
10:30–11:00 A.M.		
11:00–11:30 A.M.		
11:30 A.M.–12:00 P.M.		
12:00–12:30 P.M.		
12:30–1:00 P.M.		
1:00–1:30 P.M.		
1:30–2:00 P.M.		
2:00–2:30 P.M.		
2:30–3:00 P.M.		
3:00–3:30 P.M.		
3:30–4:00 P.M.		
4:00–4:30 P.M.		
4:30–5:00 P.M.		
5:00–5:30 P.M.		
5:30–6:00 P.M.		
6:00–6:30 P.M.		
6:30–7:00 P.M.		
7:00–7:30 P.M.		
7:30–8:00 P.M.		
8:00–8:30 P.M.		
8:30–9:00 P.M.		
9:00–9:30 P.M.		
9:30–10:00 P.M.		
10:00–10:30 P.M.		
10:30–11:00 P.M.		
11:00–11:30 P.M.		
11:30 P.M.–12:00 A.M.		

M T W TH F SA SU		Pleasurable? 1 (least) – 4 (most)
6:00–6:30 A.M.		
6:30–7:00 A.M.		
7:00–7:30 A.M.		
7:30–8:00 A.M.		
8:00–8:30 A.M.		
8:30–9:00 A.M.		
9:00–9:30 A.M.		
9:30–10:00 A.M.		
10:00–10:30 A.M.		
10:30–11:00 A.M.		
11:00–11:30 A.M.		
11:30 A.M.–12:00 P.M.		
12:00–12:30 P.M.		
12:30–1:00 P.M.		
1:00–1:30 P.M.		
1:30–2:00 P.M.		
2:00–2:30 P.M.		
2:30–3:00 P.M.		
3:00–3:30 P.M.		
3:30–4:00 P.M.		
4:00–4:30 P.M.		
4:30–5:00 P.M.		
5:00–5:30 P.M.		
5:30–6:00 P.M.		
6:00–6:30 P.M.		
6:30–7:00 P.M.		
7:00–7:30 P.M.		
7:30–8:00 P.M.		
8:00–8:30 P.M.		
8:30–9:00 P.M.		
9:00–9:30 P.M.		
9:30–10:00 P.M.		
10:00–10:30 P.M.		
10:30–11:00 P.M.		
11:00–11:30 P.M.		
11:30 P.M.–12:00 A.M.		

M T W TH F SA SU		Pleasurable? 1 (least) – 4 (most)
6:00–6:30 A.M.		
6:30–7:00 A.M.		
7:00–7:30 A.M.		
7:30–8:00 A.M.		
8:00–8:30 A.M.		
8:30–9:00 A.M.		
9:00–9:30 A.M.		
9:30–10:00 A.M.		
10:00–10:30 A.M.		
10:30–11:00 A.M.		
11:00–11:30 A.M.		
11:30 A.M.–12:00 P.M.		
12:00–12:30 P.M.		
12:30–1:00 P.M.		
1:00–1:30 P.M.		
1:30–2:00 P.M.		
2:00–2:30 P.M.		
2:30–3:00 P.M.		
3:00–3:30 P.M.		
3:30–4:00 P.M.		
4:00–4:30 P.M.		
4:30–5:00 P.M.		
5:00–5:30 P.M.		
5:30–6:00 P.M.		
6:00–6:30 P.M.		
6:30–7:00 P.M.		
7:00–7:30 P.M.		
7:30–8:00 P.M.		
8:00–8:30 P.M.		
8:30–9:00 P.M.		
9:00–9:30 P.M.		
9:30–10:00 P.M.		
10:00–10:30 P.M.		
10:30–11:00 P.M.		
11:00–11:30 P.M.		
11:30 P.M.–12:00 A.M.		

M T W TH F SA SU		Pleasurable? 1 (least) – 4 (most)
6:00–6:30 A.M.		
6:30–7:00 A.M.		
7:00–7:30 A.M.		
7:30–8:00 A.M.		
8:00–8:30 A.M.		
8:30–9:00 A.M.		
9:00–9:30 A.M.		
9:30–10:00 A.M.		
10:00–10:30 A.M.		
10:30–11:00 A.M.		
11:00–11:30 A.M.		
11:30 A.M.–12:00 P.M.		
12:00–12:30 P.M.		
12:30–1:00 P.M.		
1:00–1:30 P.M.		
1:30–2:00 P.M.		
2:00–2:30 P.M.		
2:30–3:00 P.M.		
3:00–3:30 P.M.		
3:30–4:00 P.M.		
4:00–4:30 P.M.		
4:30–5:00 P.M.		
5:00–5:30 P.M.		
5:30–6:00 P.M.		
6:00–6:30 P.M.		
6:30–7:00 P.M.		
7:00–7:30 P.M.		
7:30–8:00 P.M.		
8:00–8:30 P.M.		
8:30–9:00 P.M.		
9:00–9:30 P.M.		
9:30–10:00 P.M.		
10:00–10:30 P.M.		
10:30–11:00 P.M.		
11:00–11:30 P.M.		
11:30 P.M.–12:00 A.M.		

M T W TH F SA SU		Pleasurable? 1 (least) – 4 (most)
6:00–6:30 A.M.		
6:30–7:00 A.M.		
7:00–7:30 A.M.		
7:30–8:00 A.M.		
8:00–8:30 A.M.		
8:30–9:00 A.M.		
9:00–9:30 A.M.		
9:30–10:00 A.M.		
10:00–10:30 A.M.		
10:30–11:00 A.M.		
11:00–11:30 A.M.		
11:30 A.M.–12:00 P.M.		
12:00–12:30 P.M.		
12:30–1:00 P.M.		
1:00–1:30 P.M.		
1:30–2:00 P.M.		
2:00–2:30 P.M.		
2:30–3:00 P.M.		
3:00–3:30 P.M.		
3:30–4:00 P.M.		
4:00–4:30 P.M.		
4:30–5:00 P.M.		
5:00–5:30 P.M.		
5:30–6:00 P.M.		
6:00–6:30 P.M.		
6:30–7:00 P.M.		
7:00–7:30 P.M.		
7:30–8:00 P.M.		
8:00–8:30 P.M.		
8:30–9:00 P.M.		
9:00–9:30 P.M.		
9:30–10:00 P.M.		
10:00–10:30 P.M.		
10:30–11:00 P.M.		
11:00–11:30 P.M.		
11:30 P.M.–12:00 A.M.		

Review the Results

Congratulations on completing the challenging monitoring exercise! Now that you have finished the monitoring forms, it's time to think about what you learned about yourself as a result of doing the exercise. As you look at your forms, try to determine whether particular patterns of behavior are evident.

EXERCISE: WHAT DO YOUR DIARIES SHOW?

Do you notice any tendencies to do certain things at particular times during the day? Write down three things you noticed about how you engaged in certain activities at specific times during the day.

1. _____

2. _____

3. _____

In terms of how you thought of yourself before completing this exercise, are you engaging in more or fewer activities than you would have expected? (Circle one.)

MORE   FEWER

If you are like some people (including Robert), you may be engaging in a wide variety of activities. However, as you already know, simply engaging in many activities does not necessarily mean you will not be depressed or anxious. In fact, as you will learn shortly, it's not about the *quantity* of behaviors you engage in, but rather the *quality* of behaviors, or how much your behaviors provide you with a sense of reward and are consistent with your life values. If the quality of your behaviors has diminished substantially and you do not feel rewarded for engaging in certain life experiences, the end result can be substantial feelings of depression and anxiety.

As you further review your monitoring exercise, what were your ratings like? List the four (different) behaviors that had the highest pleasure ratings.

1. _____

2. _____

3. _____

4. _____

Why were these behaviors more rewarding than others? What is it about these activities or behaviors that make them so enjoyable?

_____

_____

Which behaviors and activities were less rewarding? List the four (different) behaviors that had the lowest pleasure ratings.

1. _____

2. _____

3. _____

4. _____

What is it about these activities or behaviors that made them so much less pleasurable than the others?

_____

_____

_____

As you review your weekly activities and ratings, what do you think might be missing from your life? What experiences or activities could have made the week more rewarding and enjoyable for you?

_____

_____

_____

Think about why you didn't engage in these activities. Was the inability to do these things in some way related to anxiety or fear?

_____

_____

_____

Finally, if you recall the eleven areas of avoidance from chapter 4, are there specific life areas (and behaviors) that you have avoided more than others? What areas are these?

_____

_____

_____

In completing the daily monitoring exercise, you should have learned a fair amount about your lifestyle, your behaviors, how you spend your time, and which behaviors are more or less pleasurable. Having this knowledge will enable you to move forward with the important behavioral changes that will need to be made to improve your mood.

WEEK 2: YOUR ENVIRONMENT, YOUR LIFE GOALS, AND YOUR ILLNESS

Now that you have a better understanding of how you spend your time and have learned that the behaviors you engage in have an impact on your mood, it's time to focus on learning more about how you can reduce feelings of anxiety and depression by changing your environment and the ways that you spend your time. During this second week, there are three specific goals to be accomplished, in the following order:

1. Learn how to create a healthier environment through understanding how the emotions of depression and anxiety can be rewarded and then to eliminate these rewards to make it less likely that your depression and anxiety will continue.

2. Identify the importance of various areas of your life and establish specific life goals that you can use as a basis for behavioral activation.

3. Begin to confront cancer and decrease your anxiety through learning how to face the experience of being diagnosed with and living with cancer and decreasing avoidance.

Creating a Healthier Environment

The first goal of this week is to continue to gather information about the extent to which you are engaging in depressed and anxious behaviors (things like passivity, avoidance of situations, staying in bed, and so on) and how people and events in your life may contribute to your depressed and anxious behavior. So the focus is on continuing to work toward creating an environment and experiences that support healthy behavior.

To create this kind of behavior, it is important that you understand that all behavior occurs for one of two reasons, or in some cases both reasons: (a) to obtain something positive or (b) to avoid or to escape something negative. For example, you brush your teeth because you obtain pleasant feelings in your mouth (something positive) and you avoid having to go to the dentist to have a cavity filled (something negative). As another example, you eat dinner because it feels good to fill your stomach and also to obtain essential vitamins and minerals. You also avoid the unpleasant feeling of being hungry, or even worse, starving. More related to the experience of cancer, you undergo treatment for cancer (surgery, radiation therapy, chemotherapy, etc.) so that you can obtain better health and avoid feeling more ill and potentially even dying. When you think about it, all of our behaviors can be understood in this way. We behave to obtain something positive, avoid something negative, or both.

EXERCISE: UNDERSTANDING WHY YOU DO WHAT YOU DO

Think of one of your behaviors—that is, anything you say or do that is observable to other people. What is this behavior?

_____

Now, write down what you think you obtain and avoid by engaging in this behavior.

OBTAIN:

_____

_____

AVOID:

_____

_____

When you think about your depressed and anxious behaviors, it might be clear what you avoid by behaving in a depressed or anxious way. For example, when you're being passive, you may be avoiding circumstances that might make you feel uncomfortable. Because of your feelings of depression, you may avoid situations that you think will be difficult to tolerate because of your mood. Such situations might include spending time with friends, going to work, going to church, and so forth. Unfortunately, when you avoid these situations, this usually makes you feel worse rather than better. This is what is referred to as a _depression feedback loop_ (Addis and Martell 2004). For example, as you look at this depression feedback loop, think about how, when you are feeling depressed, you are going to be less likely to do things that bring you a sense of pleasure, such as socializing with people, working, and going to church. Then also think about how reducing these behaviors is going to result in a worsening of depressive feelings, which will make it even less likely that you will once again engage in those behaviors. Indeed, this is a vicious cycle that must be broken if you are going to overcome your depression.

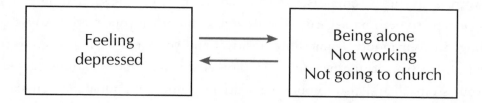

Similarly, when you have problems with anxiety, these symptoms usually occur in specific situations. Because you are anxious in these situations, it is tempting to avoid them so you can avoid feeling anxious. For example, if you have social anxiety, you may avoid being around strangers, speaking in public, or being in crowded places. If you are anxious about hearing medical feedback from your doctor, you may avoid making appointments or not show up for the ones you have scheduled.

Again, although this avoidance may create temporary relief in that you do not have to face difficult situations, the long-term consequences can be severe. If you avoid social situations and doctor's appointments, you will never be able to overcome your social anxiety and may have significant medical problems go undetected. Only through approaching these situations can you learn to be comfortable in social situations and overcome your fear of having a medical problem. This continuum is illustrated below.

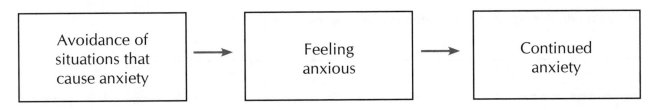

Even when you understand how depressive and anxious behaviors may be maintained by avoiding uncomfortable situations, it may be more difficult to understand how depression and anxiety can be maintained because of what you get out of it. You might be asking, "How can being depressed or anxious lead to something positive, something I'd want?" Let's think about how depressed and anxious behavior might get you something positive, at least in the short term. Maybe on some occasions, being depressed or anxious has made it easier for you to avoid certain unpleasant or stressful activities, such as chores around the house, tasks at work, having a difficult conversation with a family member or coworker, or going to that medical appointment.

Others around you may even have been willing to help you do chores or tasks if they were aware of your depressed or anxious feelings and wanted to help. Similarly, others may have been sympathetic to your avoidance of communicating or visiting the doctor, saying things such as "Don't worry about that right now. It's not your fault," "Your coworker should come to you instead of you having to approach her," or "I understand why you're afraid to go to the doctor. It's okay not to go."

Maybe at other times people have reacted in other supportive ways when you're feeling down in the dumps or anxious. For example, maybe they offer you more attention and sympathy. We're not suggesting that you deceitfully behave in a depressed or anxious way in order to get rewarded. Instead, we are simply asking you to recognize that depressed and anxious behavior sometimes can lead to positive things, which is part of the reason why you might be having trouble overcoming these emotions.

Feelings of depression or anxiety also can increase when rewards for healthy behavior decrease (for instance, when an enjoyable job starts to become stressful for some reason, or when you get into an argument with a friend or relative). So, if you put these ideas together, you can come to the conclusion that depression and anxiety and their related behaviors can happen because of (a) an increase in rewards for depressed or anxious behavior and/or (b) a decrease in rewards for healthy behavior. Therefore, by avoiding situations that provide rewards for depressed and anxious behavior and by increasing your level of positive (healthy) activities, you will have more positive thoughts and feelings, as well as a greater overall quality of life. And that is the aim of this program.

Okay, so your chances of overcoming depression and anxiety are improved when your environment supports healthy behavior and does not support depressed and anxious behavior. Some people are fortunate to have a supportive environment, but there are steps you may take to start creating such an environment if it does not already exist.

EXERCISE: CREATING A HEALTHY SOCIAL ENVIRONMENT

How do people respond to you when you are depressed or anxious?

_____

_____

_____

Can you think of specific ways your family or friends behave or react that may be helping to maintain your depressed or anxious behavior? Think carefully. When you are depressed, down, anxious, or not very active, do your friends or family members react in certain ways? Could their reactions or behaviors in some way be encouraging depressed or anxious behavior, probably unintentionally? Do they do certain things for you, speak differently to you, treat you differently?

_____

_____

_____

_____

If you believe your depressed and anxious behaviors may partially be maintained by people in your life, to begin with, you should talk with your family and friends about your need to gradually increase your healthy behaviors. Sometimes family and friends are more likely to notice your depressive behavior than your attempts at healthy behavior, but this emphasis may not be intentional. Ask them to help you with this by not focusing on your depressive or anxious symptoms but rather on your efforts to engage in more healthy alternatives. Of course, we all need support and someone to listen when life is not going well. However, the important thing to remember is to keep your depression and anxiety from being the focus of your interactions with others. For example, you might ask friends to not allow you to spend more than 20 percent of your time together talking about what is going wrong in your life to allow for more time to develop and discuss positive experiences and opportunities to engage in rewarding healthy behaviors.

Establishing Life Goals

The second goal of this week is to identify the importance of specific areas of your life and establish life goals. We think of *life goals* as those behaviors or outcomes you hope to accomplish that allow you to feel more complete as a human being, allow you to feel less anxious and depressed, build your self-esteem, and improve your quality of life. Think of where you are now in your life. Think of how you spend your time, what is important to you, what your current value system is, how your values affect your behaviors, and how other people see you. Remember that this refers to your *present self*. Now, think about the person you aspire to become. In an ideal world, how would you like to behave and how would you spend your time? Would your values be any different than they are now? Would you like to behave differently? Would you like others to view you differently? The answers to these questions represent your *ideal self*, or the person you would like to become and the behaviors that you would like to achieve. The process of behavioral activation involves moving you along this path from your perceived self toward your ideal self. It is this process that will enable you to overcome feelings of depression and anxiety. As part of this movement, your next step is to become more aware of particular activities and behaviors that may increase your pleasant experiences and sense of accomplishment, and thereby decrease symptoms of depression and anxiety.

So the next step in activating your behaviors involves focusing more specifically on some life areas that you have already begun to explore. As you focus on these different life areas and work toward establishing life goals, it will be extremely helpful for you to once again review the Cancer and the Quality of Your Life exercise (chapter 1) and Measuring the Extent of Your Avoidance exercise (chapter 4). Knowing what areas of your life might need some work and understanding some of the problematic avoidance that you might be exhibiting will help you to target areas in need of improvement.

So, as you go through this next exercise, focus on further developing an understanding of (a) how important these different areas are to you and (b) what your short- and long-term goals are in these areas.

EXERCISE: LIFE-GOAL ASSESSMENT

In the following exercise, keeping in mind the issues that are important for improving your quality of life and recalling those aspects of your life that you may be avoiding, write down what you would like to accomplish in each of the areas. Try to be as specific as possible. Also remember your behavioral monitoring exercise earlier in this chapter, and recall important experiences that may currently be missing in your life. At this point, it's unnecessary to identify specific behaviors that you will engage in to accomplish these goals. For example, you may identify a primary goal as wanting to become a better wife or husband. That is a very acceptable goal. Next week you will identify and target behaviors to help you achieve this and other important goals. For now, just describe goals that you would like to accomplish in these areas.

1. **Family relationships.** What type of brother/sister, son/daughter, father/mother do you want to be? What are your strengths? Weaknesses? Which relationships would you like to improve? What

qualities are important in close family relationships? What might you be able to do to make the relationships better?

_____

_____

_____

2. **Social relationships.** What would an ideal friendship be like for you? Are certain relationships poor at the moment? What are your strengths and limitations as a friend? What areas could be improved in your relationships with your friends? Do you have enough friends?

_____

_____

_____

3. **Romantic relationships.** What would your role be in a romantic relationship? Are you currently involved in this type of relationship, or would you like to be? If you are in a romantic relationship, how could it become better or more fulfilling?

_____

_____

_____

4. **Education/training/learning.** Would you like to pursue further education or receive specialized training? What would you like to learn more about?

_____

_____

_____

5. **Employment/career.** What type of work would you like to do? What kind of worker would you like to be? Do you enjoy work, or do you want to do something different?

_____

_____

_____

6. **Hobbies/recreation/leisure.** What hobbies and recreational activities are you currently involved with? Are there any special interests you would like to pursue or new activities you would like to experience?

_____

_____

7. **Volunteer work/charity/political activities.** What contribution would you like to make to the larger community? Are certain organizations important to you? Do you currently do any volunteer work? Would you like to?

_____

_____

_____

8. **Physical/health issues.** Do you wish to improve your diet, sleep, or exercise habits? Should you lose some weight? Should you be more compliant with cancer treatment?

_____

_____

_____

9. **Spirituality.** What, if anything, does spirituality mean to you? Are you satisfied with this area of your life? Would you like to become more spiritual?

_____

_____

_____

10. **Mental health issues.** Remembering chapter 4, do you avoid certain situations because of fear or anxiety? Would you like to face these situations? Do you need to relax more?

_____

_____

_____

In completing this life-goal assessment, you should have a much clearer picture of your ideal self and the behavioral changes you will need to make to become this person. These life goals will be central in identifying the specific behaviors and activities you will focus on in the upcoming weeks.

Confronting Your Experience with Cancer

The last goal for this week will be to begin your work toward confronting and exposing yourself to the experience of being diagnosed with and living with cancer. Through exposing yourself to situations that have caused you anxiety, such as being diagnosed with cancer, you can substantially reduce negative emotions. When you are anxious about something, the natural human tendency is to escape from and eventually avoid what is causing you to become anxious (remember the problem with avoidance discussed in chapter 4). Although this coping strategy is an understandable reaction to threatening or anxiety-provoking situations, it prevents you from learning that certain situations, events, people, sensations, or fears may be less problematic or less threatening than you are imagining.

The process of *behavioral exposure* refers to the process of exposing yourself or coming into contact with whatever situations or events cause you anxiety. When feared situations are repeatedly experienced, new evidence can be gathered that allows you to think about the situations in different ways. For example, if you have learned to be anxious about attending doctor's appointments because of your experience of being diagnosed with cancer, you may be avoiding attending future appointments. However, the more often you attend these appointments and learn that you will not be diagnosed with cancer (or another medical problem) every time you go, over time, the fear of attending appointments will decrease. Therefore, you can look at the experience of going to the doctor more realistically.

On the other hand, when people try to avoid the experiences and thoughts associated with living with cancer (for example, beliefs and attitudes associated with cancer and living with a cancer diagnosis), this tendency to avoid may actually have the paradoxical effect of increasing the intensity of anxiety. In fact, there is a good deal of research that suggests the tendency to try to avoid feared or unwanted thoughts and feelings, a process called *thought suppression*, actually increases rather than decreases problems with anxiety (Koster et al. 2003). In other words, sometimes people are worse off when they fight to forget about cancer or distract themselves from thinking about cancer.

Exposure to and acceptance of your illness is an important process toward gaining improved mental and physical health. Remember the quicksand metaphor that we described in the first chapter. Much as fighting and struggling when stuck in quicksand may actually worsen the situation and cause you to sink faster, sometimes fighting with your thoughts and trying to force them out of consciousness isn't the best approach either. Instead, accepting and trying to understand and relax may be a more optimal approach.

So as the final exercise for this week, the goal is to work toward beginning this process of experiencing and accepting for the purpose of overcoming your anxiety and fear.

EXERCISE: EXPERIENCING A CANCER DIAGNOSIS

Without referring back to chapter 1 where you completed a similar exercise, please write about your experience of being diagnosed with cancer. For you to be able to overcome your fears and anxieties, it is important that you repeatedly expose yourself to anxiety-provoking experiences, and this is the goal in repeating this task. Just write about the specific day that you were diagnosed with cancer. Please write in the first person (using "I") and in the present tense (as though you have actually just heard from a medical professional that you have cancer). Describe the event in as much detail as possible, including what you are seeing, what you are hearing, what your specific thoughts and fears are, and what emotional experiences you are having. There is no requirement for length. Just write as much as you need to fully describe this experience.

_____

_____

_____

_____

_____

_____

_____

_____

_____

When you have finished this exercise, take a moment to reflect. What was your experience like as you completed the exercise? As you look back at chapter 1, how similar or different was what you wrote? What emotions did you feel? Were they unwanted? Were they unwanted but in some way helpful, healing, or therapeutic? How was it different from trying to avoid the thoughts or experiences associated with being diagnosed with cancer? Was your experience more tolerable than the first time you completed the exercise? Was it less anxiety provoking? Remember, in the weeks to follow, that exposure to, understanding of, and acceptance of anxiety- or depression-provoking experiences are important components of improved physical and mental health.

WEEK 3: ACTIVITY IDENTIFICATION, BEHAVIORAL ACTIVATION, AND CONFRONTING CANCER

Now that you have learned to explore your value system and goals as they relate to important areas in your life, it's time to take more specific steps toward developing a new behavioral pattern that will allow you better access to pleasurable and rewarding life experiences. For this third week, there are three major goals, in the following order:

1. Establish observable and measurable target activities that are consistent with your Life-Goal Assessment. Establish the difficulty of completing identified activities.

2. Engage in the process of behavioral activation by designing a Master Activity Log and a Behavior Checkout, and by beginning to activate.

3. Continue to confront cancer through behavioral exposure.

Establishing Observable and Measurable Target Behaviors

Now that you have determined the importance of various life areas and life goals that you would like to work toward, it's time to start focusing on how to achieve particular goals. The primary strategy for doing this will be to examine your goals and to identify actual behaviors or activities that will help you to achieve these goals. In completing this exercise, sometimes you might identify clusters of activities that make up larger long-term goals. For example, a long-term goal of getting a college degree might include specific actions such as getting information on various academic programs, meeting with college advisors, saving money to purchase text-books and pay for tuition, enrolling in classes, and studying several hours per week. As another example, a long-term goal of developing a closer relationship with a family member may include specific actions such as spending more time together, engaging in more activities that would bring about mutual enjoyment, offering to babysit her/his child, contacting each other at least once per week on the phone, initiating e-mail contact, or developing more useful strategies to resolve conflict in the relationship. Identifying and engaging in a cluster of activities aimed at a specific long-term goal will be satisfying, but it's important to remember that the achievement of a long-term goal will take time, and patience will sometimes be very important. That is why it will also be important to identify behaviors and activities that will bring you a more immediate experience of pleasure, reward, or satisfaction.

In addition to selecting activities and behaviors that involve both short- and long-term rewards, it will be extremely important to select activities across a wide range of the life areas that are important to you. Sometimes people have a tendency to put too much emphasis on one aspect of their lives at the expense of other important areas. For example, recall from earlier in this chapter the substantial amount of time that Robert was engaging in work activities at the expense of other important life areas and how this overemphasis resulted in increased depression. As another example, consider someone who is in a romantic relationship and sacrifices all their time and energy for this other person. Although it is clearly important to make sacrifices for someone you love, there is a danger in being overly enmeshed with someone to the extent that you completely define yourself by that relationship. If you do this, when the relationship is not going well or even ends, you may have the experience of feeling as though you have nothing else, that you have lost everything. That is why it is important to define yourself through many life roles and behaviors. When one aspect of your life is unsatisfactory, other important and rewarding experiences can still occur, decreasing the likelihood that you will feel depressed or anxious. So when you are selecting activities, keep in mind the importance of selecting activities and behaviors from a variety of life areas.

Finally, when you are selecting your behaviors, make sure to set reasonable goals that are attainable given your diagnosis of cancer. For example, if you are in the midst of radiation therapy or chemotherapy and are experiencing significant side effects that may include fatigue and nausea, it would be unreasonable to think about setting high standards for an exercise routine. Indeed, rather than planning on walking, jogging, or cycling, at this stage it would be more reasonable to establish a goal of getting out of bed to accomplish a household task or chore that might involve some physical exertion. Then, when you feel more capable physically, you can modify goals and behaviors to better meet your long-term goals for an exercise program.

GUIDELINES FOR SELECTING ACTIVITIES

In general, if you believe that completing a particular activity or behavior will bring you a sense of pleasure or accomplishment, and the behavior is reasonable given where you are with your cancer diagnosis, then it probably would be good to include it. When selecting activities, it is important to remember that they must have two specific characteristics. They must be both observable by others and measurable. Therefore, general goals like "thinking more positively" or "building my self-esteem" would not be the best choices. The reason they don't work as well is because other people cannot see you think differently nor build your self-esteem. They are also less preferred because they cannot be measured. In other words, you cannot say precisely how many times you will accomplish these behaviors in a given week or how long they will last.

On the other hand, goals like "spending more time with my mother" or "exercising more often" would be terrific choices. These activities could be both observable and measurable in the sense that you could meet with your mother one time per week and spend at least twenty minutes with her each time. You could also decide to engage in brisk walking for thirty minutes a day for three days out of each week. These behaviors would be good choices because other people can see you do them, and they are also measurable in the sense that you can identify how often and for how long they will occur. If these two conditions are met, you have identified suitable activities to be included in your behavioral program.

Sometimes it will be tempting to select very difficult activities. Although it is good to be ambitious and to challenge yourself, try to make sure you select activities across a range of difficulty, with only a few being more difficult, long-term behaviors or activities. In fact, to improve the likelihood of initial success and to ease your transition into the behavioral activation program, make sure that a couple of activities you select will be relatively easy to accomplish. For example, if you are used to sleeping until 10:00 A.M. and are finding that you have a shortage of time during the day, you may want to select the activity of getting out of bed before 9:00 A.M. five days a week. Note that this behavior is both observable and measurable and thus okay for inclusion in your program.

DECIDING ON ACTIVITIES

Now that you understand which behaviors are best to include, it's time to work on identifying specific behaviors that will form the basis for your behavioral activation. Using the Activity Difficulty Assessment Form below, brainstorm about activities and behaviors that would be useful for accomplishing the goals you have outlined. To help you with this process, make sure to refer to the avoidance patterns that you identified in chapter 4. As avoidance can be extremely problematic in your life, if you identified areas that you were avoiding, perhaps out of fear or anxiety, it probably would be good to include activities and behaviors that allowed you to approach these situations. For example, if you were avoiding an interaction with a friend because of a recent argument, you might want to include contacting this friend as an important activity. Second, remember the daily monitoring assignment you completed in week one, when you identified current patterns of behaving and highlighted important behaviors that you were not engaging in. Third, make sure to use the Life-Goal Assessment from last week as the basis for selecting behaviors, remembering to select activities and behaviors from a range of life areas, to increase the breadth of satisfaction and reward in your life. Fourth, now is the time to consider whether it will be useful to include the supplemental behavioral strategies outlined later in this workbook (chapters 6 through 10). If you are having difficulties with medication management, solving problems in your life, poor sleep, social problems or difficulties communicating, or problems with pain and an inability to relax, these problems should be addressed in your behavioral plan. Therefore, scan through these later chapters now and decide whether you should include one or more behaviors in your hierarchy. For example, if you have difficulties with managing your medicine, "learning to manage medications" could be one of your activities. If you're having trouble sleeping, "learning to sleep more effectively" would be included. "Learning how to relax" could be another identified behavior.

In total, you should select fifteen activities that are personalized to your goals, needs, and desires. As you think about and select these potential activities, add them to the Activity Difficulty Assessment Form. Remember that the activities should be both observable and measurable and that activities should be directly relevant to the Life-Goal Assessment you completed last week. Remember that the more you can address your life goals in the formulation of activities, the more likely you will experience the activities as both pleasurable and meaningful. Once you have outlined the activities and behaviors on the Activity Difficulty Assessment Form, your next step is to rank them from 1 (easiest to accomplish) to 15 (hardest to accomplish). This step is very important, as it will dictate the order in which you will activate your behaviors. In order to make sure you have success in this program, we want you to begin the process of behavioral activation by working through some of the easier activities and behaviors and then gradually work toward some of the harder activities.

EXERCISE: ACTIVITY DIFFICULTY ASSESSMENT FORM

Compile your fifteen activities and rate the difficulty of each from 1 (least difficult) to 15 (most difficult).

ACTIVITY	RANK

Beginning the Process of Behavioral Activation

After completing your work of establishing life goals that are important to you and identifying specific observable and measurable activities and behaviors that may assist you in achieving these goals, your primary goal will be to progressively work toward accomplishing these activities. This is the beginning stage of behavioral activation, a strategy that will be useful in progressively increasing your activity level and rewarding experiences while also decreasing your depressive and anxious symptoms. To allow you to monitor your progress in activating your behaviors, the Master Activity Log and Behavior Checkout forms will be very useful.

DEVELOPING YOUR MASTER ACTIVITY LOG

Now that you have identified fifteen activities, you will need a plan for working these activities into your life and monitoring your progress. The Master Activity Log is a useful method to track your progress on a weekly basis. In the first column, beginning with the least difficult exercise, go ahead and list your activities according to the difficulty levels you established on the Activity Difficulty Assessment Form. In the next two columns, fill in your "Ideal Goal" for each activity, including: (a) the number of days you eventually would like to complete the activity in a one-week period [indicated by a "# "] and (b) the duration of the activity, indicated by the word "Time." You may write "UF" if the goal is for the activity to continue "until finished." This would be an appropriate goal if the task was something like "making your bed," "attending a church service," or "speaking to a potential employer about a job opportunity." In all cases, it would make little sense to time the behavior or stop it before it was completed.

Remember to challenge yourself without becoming overwhelmed and to set reasonable goals. As indicated on the sample Master Activity Log below, for each activity identified, find the column marked "Goal" and write down the number of times you will eventually engage in the activity ("#") and for how long ("Time"). For example, as illustrated on the sample Master Activity Log, this patient specified the frequency and duration of time that he ultimately desired to engage in each of his target behaviors. As you can see, on a weekly basis, this patient progressively increased the number of activities that he was to engage in, and on a week-to-week basis was largely successful in meeting his goals. As you move through each week of behavioral activation, you too will progressively add more activities to your Behavior Checkout (explained below) and the results of your weekly progress will be recorded on the Master Activity Log.

SAMPLE MASTER ACTIVITY LOG

Activity	Ideal Goal #	Ideal Goal Time	Week 3 Goal #	Week 3 Goal Time	Week 3 Do Time	Week 3 Do	Week 4 Goal #	Week 4 Goal Time	Week 4 Do Time	Week 4 Do	Week 5 Goal #	Week 5 Goal Time	Week 5 Do Time	Week 5 Do	Week 6 Goal #	Week 6 Goal Time	Week 6 Do Time	Week 6 Do
GO TO WORK	5	UF	5	UF	UF	5	5	UF	UF	5	5	UF	UF	5	5	UF	UF	5
WAKE UP BY 9 A.M.	7	UF	6	UF	UF	7	7	UF	UF	7	7	UF	UF	7	7	UF	UF	7
PLAY WITH THE DOG	7	30 m	5	20 m		7	7	30 m	30 m	7	7	30 m	30 m	7	7	30 m	30 m	7
MAKE DINNER	3	UF					2	UF	UF	3	3	UF	UF	3	3	UF	UF	3
WASH DISHES	6	UF					3	UF	UF	2	3	UF	UF	1	2	UF	UF	2
CALL FRIENDS/FAMILY	2	UF													2	UF	UF	3
BRISK WALK	5	30 m													3	15 m	15 m	2
GARDENING	4	60 m																
KNIT OR CROCHET	3	60 m																
VISIT FRIEND	1	45 m																
LETTER TO FRIEND	1	UF																
GO TO SENIOR CENTER	2	UF																
ATTEND CHURCH	1	UF																

EXERCISE: YOUR MASTER ACTIVITY LOG

Activity	Ideal Goal #	Time	Week 1 Goal #	Time	Do	Week 2 Goal #	Time	Do	Week 3 Goal #	Time	Do	Week 4 Goal #	Time	Do

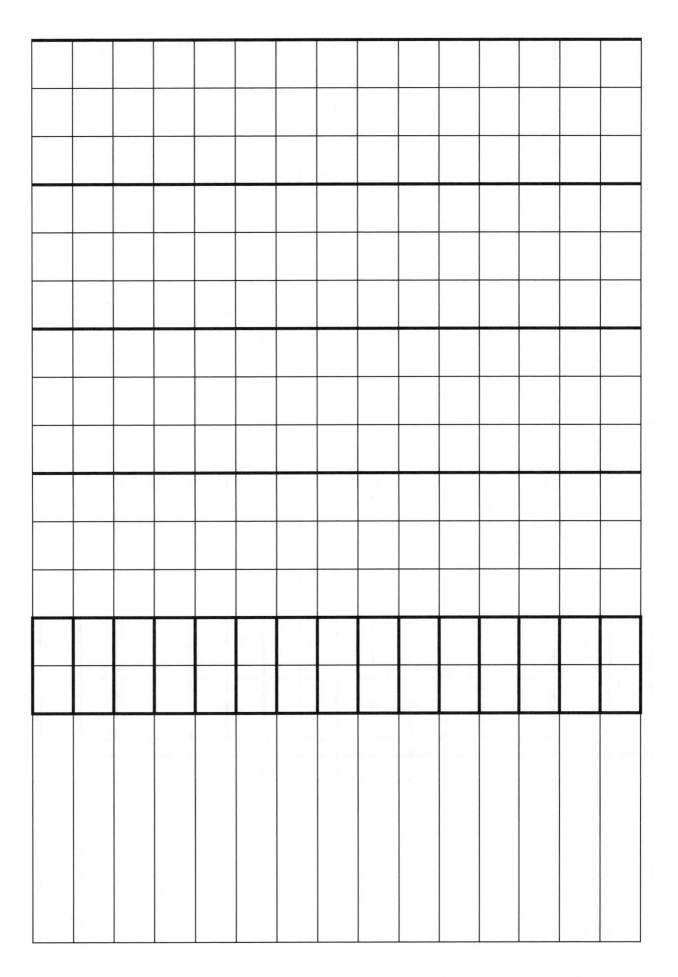

Activity	Ideal Goal		Week ___ 5			Week ___ 6			Week ___ 7			Week ___ 8		
	#	Time	Goal		Do	Goal		Do	Goal		Do	Goal		Do
			#	Time		#	Time		#	Time		#	Time	

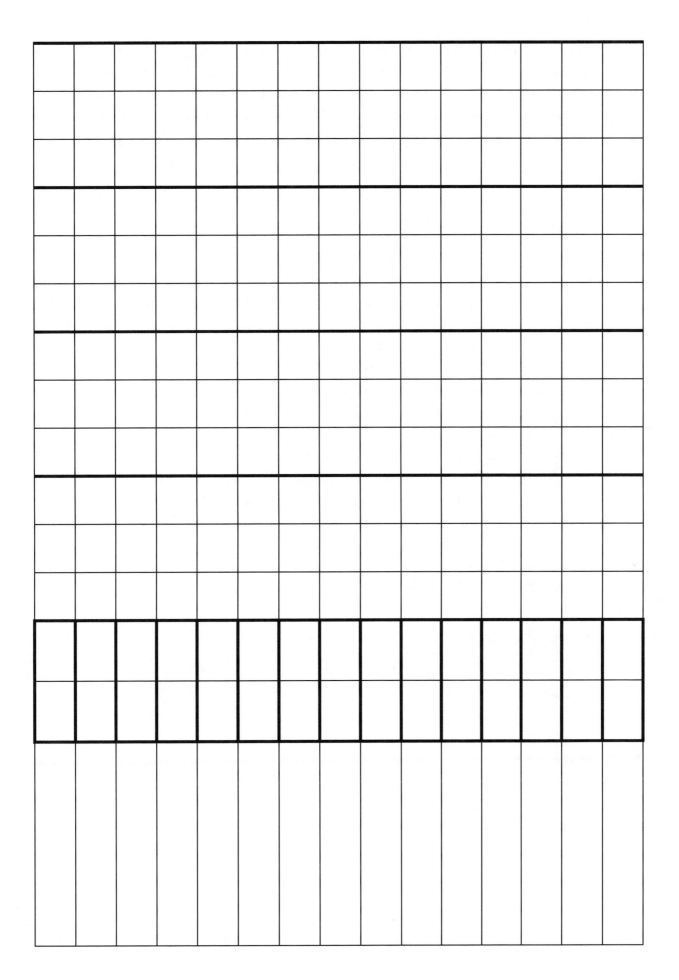

As you can see from the sample Master Activity Log, you will engage in the process of activating your behaviors over the course of the next eight weeks (and hopefully long after you have completed this workbook). Keep in mind that over the next several weeks you should consider setting a weekly goal that is less than the "Ideal Goal" and then slowly increasing the goal for that activity in future weeks until you have reached the "Ideal Goal." For this first week, only chart the first three to four activities on your list. The second week, add two or three more, and so on.

THE BEHAVIOR CHECKOUT

For each of the eight weeks that you are engaging in behavioral activation, you are going to chart your activities on what is referred to as a Behavior Checkout. This form will be useful for recording your progress on a daily basis, whereas the Master Activity Log will be completed at the end of each week. A sample Behavior Checkout is completed below. For this first week, you are going to start off by monitoring the first three or four behaviors on your Master Activity Log. So go ahead and write down these behaviors on your week 1 Behavior Checkout, along with the number of times you will engage in each of these behaviors over the next week (in the "#" column) and the length of time you will spend in each activity (remember that some will be "UF"—"until finished." For each day, over this next week, circle "Y" if you completed the activity and "N" if you did not. To ensure that you maintain accurate records, it is best if you set aside a specific time of the day to complete this task (perhaps before bedtime). Once you have completed the goals for the week, you may circle "G." Circling "G" indicates that you have successfully met your goal for the week. After circling "G," you no longer need to worry about engaging in that behavior any further, although you may if you wish. Also remember that you don't have to work toward other behaviors on your Master Activity Log, although if you'd like to, that's okay. You will address these other behaviors in future weeks.

SAMPLE BEHAVIOR CHECKOUT

Behavior Checkout—Week 4

Activity	#	Time	Monday	Tuesday	Wednesday	Thursday	Friday	Saturday	Sunday
Go to work	5	UF	Y (N) G	(Y) N G	(Y) N G	Y (N) G	(Y) N G	(Y) N G	(Y) N G
Wake by 9 A.M.	7	UF	(Y) N G	(Y) N G	(Y) N G	(Y) N G	(Y) N G	(Y) N G	(Y) N G
Play with dog	7	30 min	(Y) N G	(Y) N G	(Y) N G	(Y) N G	(Y) N G	(Y) N G	(Y) N G
Make dinner	2	UF	(Y) N G	Y (N) G	Y (N) G	(Y) N (G)	Y (N) G	(Y) N (G)	Y (N) G
Wash dishes	3	UF	Y (N) G	Y (N) G	(Y) N G	Y (N) G	(Y) N G	Y (N) G	Y (N) G
			Y N G	Y N G	Y N G	Y N G	Y N G	Y N G	Y N G
			Y N G	Y N G	Y N G	Y N G	Y N G	Y N G	Y N G
			Y N G	Y N G	Y N G	Y N G	Y N G	Y N G	Y N G
			Y N G	Y N G	Y N G	Y N G	Y N G	Y N G	Y N G
			Y N G	Y N G	Y N G	Y N G	Y N G	Y N G	Y N G
			Y N G	Y N G	Y N G	Y N G	Y N G	Y N G	Y N G
			Y N G	Y N G	Y N G	Y N G	Y N G	Y N G	Y N G

MY WEEKLY BEHAVIOR CHECKOUT
Week 1

Activity	#	Time	Monday	Tuesday	Wednesday	Thursday	Friday	Saturday	Sunday
			Y N G	Y N G	Y N G	Y N G	Y N G	Y N G	Y N G
			Y N G	Y N G	Y N G	Y N G	Y N G	Y N G	Y N G
			Y N G	Y N G	Y N G	Y N G	Y N G	Y N G	Y N G
			Y N G	Y N G	Y N G	Y N G	Y N G	Y N G	Y N G
			Y N G	Y N G	Y N G	Y N G	Y N G	Y N G	Y N G
			Y N G	Y N G	Y N G	Y N G	Y N G	Y N G	Y N G
			Y N G	Y N G	Y N G	Y N G	Y N G	Y N G	Y N G
			Y N G	Y N G	Y N G	Y N G	Y N G	Y N G	Y N G
			Y N G	Y N G	Y N G	Y N G	Y N G	Y N G	Y N G
			Y N G	Y N G	Y N G	Y N G	Y N G	Y N G	Y N G
			Y N G	Y N G	Y N G	Y N G	Y N G	Y N G	Y N G
			Y N G	Y N G	Y N G	Y N G	Y N G	Y N G	Y N G
			Y N G	Y N G	Y N G	Y N G	Y N G	Y N G	Y N G
			Y N G	Y N G	Y N G	Y N G	Y N G	Y N G	Y N G
			Y N G	Y N G	Y N G	Y N G	Y N G	Y N G	Y N G
			Y N G	Y N G	Y N G	Y N G	Y N G	Y N G	Y N G

A Cancer Patient's Guide to Overcoming Depression & Anxiety

MY WEEKLY BEHAVIOR CHECKOUT
Week 2

Activity	#	Time	Monday	Tuesday	Wednesday	Thursday	Friday	Saturday	Sunday
			Y N G	Y N G	Y N G	Y N G	Y N G	Y N G	Y N G
			Y N G	Y N G	Y N G	Y N G	Y N G	Y N G	Y N G
			Y N G	Y N G	Y N G	Y N G	Y N G	Y N G	Y N G
			Y N G	Y N G	Y N G	Y N G	Y N G	Y N G	Y N G
			Y N G	Y N G	Y N G	Y N G	Y N G	Y N G	Y N G
			Y N G	Y N G	Y N G	Y N G	Y N G	Y N G	Y N G
			Y N G	Y N G	Y N G	Y N G	Y N G	Y N G	Y N G
			Y N G	Y N G	Y N G	Y N G	Y N G	Y N G	Y N G
			Y N G	Y N G	Y N G	Y N G	Y N G	Y N G	Y N G
			Y N G	Y N G	Y N G	Y N G	Y N G	Y N G	Y N G
			Y N G	Y N G	Y N G	Y N G	Y N G	Y N G	Y N G
			Y N G	Y N G	Y N G	Y N G	Y N G	Y N G	Y N G
			Y N G	Y N G	Y N G	Y N G	Y N G	Y N G	Y N G

MY WEEKLY BEHAVIOR CHECKOUT
Week 3

Activity	#	Time	Monday	Tuesday	Wednesday	Thursday	Friday	Saturday	Sunday
			Y N G	Y N G	Y N G	Y N G	Y N G	Y N G	Y N G
			Y N G	Y N G	Y N G	Y N G	Y N G	Y N G	Y N G
			Y N G	Y N G	Y N G	Y N G	Y N G	Y N G	Y N G
			Y N G	Y N G	Y N G	Y N G	Y N G	Y N G	Y N G
			Y N G	Y N G	Y N G	Y N G	Y N G	Y N G	Y N G
			Y N G	Y N G	Y N G	Y N G	Y N G	Y N G	Y N G
			Y N G	Y N G	Y N G	Y N G	Y N G	Y N G	Y N G
			Y N G	Y N G	Y N G	Y N G	Y N G	Y N G	Y N G
			Y N G	Y N G	Y N G	Y N G	Y N G	Y N G	Y N G
			Y N G	Y N G	Y N G	Y N G	Y N G	Y N G	Y N G
			Y N G	Y N G	Y N G	Y N G	Y N G	Y N G	Y N G
			Y N G	Y N G	Y N G	Y N G	Y N G	Y N G	Y N G
			Y N G	Y N G	Y N G	Y N G	Y N G	Y N G	Y N G
			Y N G	Y N G	Y N G	Y N G	Y N G	Y N G	Y N G
			Y N G	Y N G	Y N G	Y N G	Y N G	Y N G	Y N G
			Y N G	Y N G	Y N G	Y N G	Y N G	Y N G	Y N G

MY WEEKLY BEHAVIOR CHECKOUT

Week 4

Activity	#	Time	Monday	Tuesday	Wednesday	Thursday	Friday	Saturday	Sunday
			Y N G	Y N G	Y N G	Y N G	Y N G	Y N G	Y N G
			Y N G	Y N G	Y N G	Y N G	Y N G	Y N G	Y N G
			Y N G	Y N G	Y N G	Y N G	Y N G	Y N G	Y N G
			Y N G	Y N G	Y N G	Y N G	Y N G	Y N G	Y N G
			Y N G	Y N G	Y N G	Y N G	Y N G	Y N G	Y N G
			Y N G	Y N G	Y N G	Y N G	Y N G	Y N G	Y N G
			Y N G	Y N G	Y N G	Y N G	Y N G	Y N G	Y N G
			Y N G	Y N G	Y N G	Y N G	Y N G	Y N G	Y N G
			Y N G	Y N G	Y N G	Y N G	Y N G	Y N G	Y N G
			Y N G	Y N G	Y N G	Y N G	Y N G	Y N G	Y N G
			Y N G	Y N G	Y N G	Y N G	Y N G	Y N G	Y N G
			Y N G	Y N G	Y N G	Y N G	Y N G	Y N G	Y N G
			Y N G	Y N G	Y N G	Y N G	Y N G	Y N G	Y N G
			Y N G	Y N G	Y N G	Y N G	Y N G	Y N G	Y N G
			Y N G	Y N G	Y N G	Y N G	Y N G	Y N G	Y N G
			Y N G	Y N G	Y N G	Y N G	Y N G	Y N G	Y N G

MY WEEKLY BEHAVIOR CHECKOUT
Week 5

Activity	#	Time	Monday	Tuesday	Wednesday	Thursday	Friday	Saturday	Sunday
			Y N G	Y N G	Y N G	Y N G	Y N G	Y N G	Y N G
			Y N G	Y N G	Y N G	Y N G	Y N G	Y N G	Y N G
			Y N G	Y N G	Y N G	Y N G	Y N G	Y N G	Y N G
			Y N G	Y N G	Y N G	Y N G	Y N G	Y N G	Y N G
			Y N G	Y N G	Y N G	Y N G	Y N G	Y N G	Y N G
			Y N G	Y N G	Y N G	Y N G	Y N G	Y N G	Y N G
			Y N G	Y N G	Y N G	Y N G	Y N G	Y N G	Y N G
			Y N G	Y N G	Y N G	Y N G	Y N G	Y N G	Y N G
			Y N G	Y N G	Y N G	Y N G	Y N G	Y N G	Y N G
			Y N G	Y N G	Y N G	Y N G	Y N G	Y N G	Y N G
			Y N G	Y N G	Y N G	Y N G	Y N G	Y N G	Y N G
			Y N G	Y N G	Y N G	Y N G	Y N G	Y N G	Y N G
			Y N G		Y N G	Y N G	Y N G	Y N G	Y N G

MY WEEKLY BEHAVIOR CHECKOUT
Week 6

Activity	#	Time	Monday	Tuesday	Wednesday	Thursday	Friday	Saturday	Sunday
			Y N G	Y N G	Y N G	Y N G	Y N G	Y N G	Y N G
			Y N G	Y N G	Y N G	Y N G	Y N G	Y N G	Y N G
			Y N G	Y N G	Y N G	Y N G	Y N G	Y N G	Y N G
			Y N G	Y N G	Y N G	Y N G	Y N G	Y N G	Y N G
			Y N G	Y N G	Y N G	Y N G	Y N G	Y N G	Y N G
			Y N G	Y N G	Y N G	Y N G	Y N G	Y N G	Y N G
			Y N G	Y N G	Y N G	Y N G	Y N G	Y N G	Y N G
			Y N G	Y N G	Y N G	Y N G	Y N G	Y N G	Y N G
			Y N G	Y N G	Y N G	Y N G	Y N G	Y N G	Y N G
			Y N G	Y N G	Y N G	Y N G	Y N G	Y N G	Y N G
			Y N G	Y N G	Y N G	Y N G	Y N G	Y N G	Y N G
			Y N G	Y N G	Y N G	Y N G	Y N G	Y N G	Y N G
			Y N G	Y N G	Y N G	Y N G	Y N G	Y N G	Y N G
			Y N G	Y N G	Y N G	Y N G	Y N G	Y N G	Y N G

MY WEEKLY BEHAVIOR CHECKOUT
Week 7

Activity	#	Time	Monday	Tuesday	Wednesday	Thursday	Friday	Saturday	Sunday
			Y N G	Y N G	Y N G	Y N G	Y N G	Y N G	Y N G
			Y N G	Y N G	Y N G	Y N G	Y N G	Y N G	Y N G
			Y N G	Y N G	Y N G	Y N G	Y N G	Y N G	Y N G
			Y N G	Y N G	Y N G	Y N G	Y N G	Y N G	Y N G
			Y N G	Y N G	Y N G	Y N G	Y N G	Y N G	Y N G
			Y N G	Y N G	Y N G	Y N G	Y N G	Y N G	Y N G
			Y N G	Y N G	Y N G	Y N G	Y N G	Y N G	Y N G
			Y N G	Y N G	Y N G	Y N G	Y N G	Y N G	Y N G
			Y N G	Y N G	Y N G	Y N G	Y N G	Y N G	Y N G
			Y N G	Y N G	Y N G	Y N G	Y N G	Y N G	Y N G
			Y N G	Y N G	Y N G	Y N G	Y N G	Y N G	Y N G
			Y N G	Y N G	Y N G	Y N G	Y N G	Y N G	Y N G
			Y N G	Y N G	Y N G	Y N G	Y N G	Y N G	Y N G
			Y N G	Y N G	Y N G	Y N G	Y N G	Y N G	Y N G

MY WEEKLY BEHAVIOR CHECKOUT
Week 8

Activity	#	Time	Monday	Tuesday	Wednesday	Thursday	Friday	Saturday	Sunday
			Y N G	Y N G	Y N G	Y N G	Y N G	Y N G	Y N G
			Y N G	Y N G	Y N G	Y N G	Y N G	Y N G	Y N G
			Y N G	Y N G	Y N G	Y N G	Y N G	Y N G	Y N G
			Y N G	Y N G	Y N G	Y N G	Y N G	Y N G	Y N G
			Y N G	Y N G	Y N G	Y N G	Y N G	Y N G	Y N G
			Y N G	Y N G	Y N G	Y N G	Y N G	Y N G	Y N G
			Y N G	Y N G	Y N G	Y N G	Y N G	Y N G	Y N G
			Y N G	Y N G	Y N G	Y N G	Y N G	Y N G	Y N G
			Y N G	Y N G	Y N G	Y N G	Y N G	Y N G	Y N G
			Y N G	Y N G	Y N G	Y N G	Y N G	Y N G	Y N G
			Y N G	Y N G	Y N G	Y N G	Y N G	Y N G	Y N G
			Y N G	Y N G	Y N G	Y N G	Y N G	Y N G	Y N G
			Y N G	Y N G	Y N G	Y N G	Y N G	Y N G	Y N G
			Y N G	Y N G	Y N G	Y N G	Y N G	Y N G	Y N G

You have just completed your first week of behavioral activation. Congratulations! As you reflect on your Behavior Checkout, how difficult was it to complete your three to four activities? As you think about what you accomplished, how rewarding was it for you to engage in the behaviors? Did you feel good inside when you were doing them or immediately after completing them? Was it very difficult to complete them, and did you only experience pleasure or accomplishment after you had completed them? Did you complete them and feel no pleasure or reward at all? Your responses to these questions should be written below and will be addressed later in this chapter.

_____

_____

_____

_____

_____

_____

_____

Continuing to Confront Cancer Through Exposure

The last goal for this week will be to continue your work toward confronting and exposing yourself to the experience of living with cancer. Remember that although there are many important changes you can make to improve your life and mood after being diagnosed with cancer, acceptance of being diagnosed and treated for cancer is an important stage of gaining improved mental and physical health. Continuing with this process, for next week we would like you to do another brief writing assignment.

EXERCISE: YOUR EXPERIENCE OF LIVING WITH CANCER

Please write about your experience of living with cancer. Here you can write about how your life has progressed or changed after being diagnosed with cancer. Please write in the first person (using "I"). Describe the last few months (or several years) in as much detail as you wish, being sure to include issues surrounding your treatment, visits to your oncologist or primary care physician, how your life is better or worse now that you are living with cancer, and what specific thoughts, fears, and emotional experiences you continue to have. How has living with cancer affected your lifestyle? How have family and friends responded to your illness? What (family or peer) reactions have you been pleased with? What reactions have you been disappointed with? Again, there is no requirement for length. Just write as much as you need to fully describe this experience.

When you have finished this exercise, take a moment to reflect. What was your experience like as you completed the exercise? What emotions were experienced? Were they unwanted? Were they unwanted but in some way helpful, healing, or therapeutic? How was it different from trying to avoid the thoughts or experiences associated with living with cancer? Remember that exposure to, understanding of, and acceptance of anxiety- or depression-provoking experiences are important components of improved physical and mental health.

WEEKS 4 THROUGH 10: BEHAVIORAL ACTIVATION, RUMINATION-CUED ACTIVATION, AND CONFRONTING CANCER

Other clinicians and researchers who do behavioral activation have encouraged people to think about activating behavior as though they are conducting behavioral experiments (Addis and Martell 2001). *Behavioral experiments* refer to the idea that you develop an interest in completing certain behaviors no matter what the results might be, then assess the outcome of completing the behavior, much as a scientist would evaluate the outcome of a project he or she conducted. In your situation, the experiment involves engaging in the behaviors and evaluating how they affect your mood. Importantly, your job as a scientist involves making sure that (a) you are fully involved in your behaviors when you are doing them, (b) you avoid evaluating the outcome of your behavior while it is going on, and (c) you try your behavioral experiments more than once (Addis and Martell 2001). So work hard to really focus on your new behaviors while you are doing them. Try to eliminate all the distractions that can occur and really experience the moment of activating a behavior. Be involved and committed to what you are doing. Evaluate the experiment after it is over, thinking about whether your mood changed at any point in time while you engaged in the behavior. Finally, make sure to establish whether a behavior really does not positively affect your mood before deciding to discontinue performing the behavior. Sometimes these initial behavior changes can create anxiety. So try behaviors several times before drawing any conclusions about their usefulness toward changing your mood.

It's important to remember that change will take time. Depression and anxiety are very powerful emotions. So if you did not experience a tremendous change in your emotion after completing your behaviors last week, don't panic. This will be a process that will take time. Just as the powerful feelings of depression and anxiety probably did not develop overnight, it is unlikely that they will disappear right away. For now, we ask that you be patient. Have faith that you are engaging in a new process that could be very useful to you if you give it a chance.

If you did not meet your goals, it's important to ask yourself why. Can you think of any obstacles or problems that might have affected your ability to complete your behaviors? Were you able to manage your time appropriately throughout the week and set your behavioral goals as a high priority? If not, try to be more specific about which days (and times) you will complete your behaviors. Commit yourself to engaging in these behaviors at that time, no matter what your mood might be when the time comes. Remember that this is one of the most important lessons to be learned in behavioral activation—the notion that you can engage in certain behaviors even though you may feel like you are not in a good mood. Try to take action no matter what emotion you are experiencing. Your behaviors can be separate from your emotions. You may not feel as though you can drive your children to school, engage in some exercise, prepare a meal, converse with a friend, attend church, or go shopping. However, providing this feeling (or barrier) is an emotional one rather than a physical limitation associated with your cancer, you can overcome these feelings and still decide to act. If the barrier is primarily the result of feeling bad physically, try your best to work within your physical limitations and do the best you can—and also be sure to see your doctor to see if there is anything you can do to feel better physically.

MODIFYING WEEKLY GOALS

At the end of week 1, be sure to take your completed Behavior Checkout and use it to complete the Master Activity Log. Be sure to write down your behaviors in the left column, and record the number of times and the duration of time that you intended to engage in a particular behavior (under the "# " and "Time" columns for "Goal") as well as the actual number of times you completed these behaviors in the "Do" column of the Master Activity Log.

If you met your goals, you should probably think about slowly beginning to increase the frequency and time of the activities for the upcoming week (assuming you have not yet met your ideal goal). Also, providing you are meeting your goals on a weekly basis, you should probably think about continuing to engage in these behaviors, but also adding another behavior or two each week to work toward. If you don't meet your goals, you will want to decide whether the weekly goals were (a) reasonable and missed due to unforeseen circumstances or obstacles or (b) unreasonable and set too high. In the first situation, you could leave the same goals for the next week and address obstacles as necessary. In the second situation, you might strongly consider reducing the weekly goal (and potentially rethinking the ideal goal) to make it more manageable and increase the likelihood that you will follow through.

It should be noted that in behavioral activation, we generally do not work on developing specific "skills" in the context of treatment. Instead, the underlying belief is that most people who engage in treatment have the necessary skills to complete the behaviors that they have identified as important. We also believe that skills can be learned naturally over time as you begin to engage in your activities and with other people. However, we also recognize that there will be certain exceptions to these ideas. For example, there may be certain problematic behavioral deficits that limit your ability to complete the goals that you have identified for yourself. In such cases, additional skill-training strategies may be necessary to add to the behavioral activation treatment.

For example, it might be important to better learn how to problem solve around not being able to complete goals or how to deal with difficult situations related to your cancer, relationships, work, and other things. It also might be necessary to learn more effective social, communication, and assertiveness skills if you recognize that deficits in these areas act as barriers to completing your activities and behaviors. Other issues such as learning how to better manage your medications, how to improve your sleep, how to relax more effectively, and how to better cope with your pain also might need considerable attention. The earlier you recognize these potential problems, and the sooner you begin to act toward resolving them, the more likely you will be to experience a more rewarding lifestyle that will help you to overcome your depression and anxiety. Therefore, when you recognize that such problems may be limiting your ability to effectively change your behavior, you should take some time to work through these issues. Chapter 6 includes well-studied methods that will help you to overcome these problems and includes suggestions on whether these additional strategies should be incorporated into your treatment.

GOALS FOR WEEKS 4 THROUGH 10

In the next several weeks, there are three important goals for you to focus on. First, as you have already come to understand, you will need to continue to engage in the process of behavioral activation. For each week, continue to design your Behavior Checkout and modify goals as per the guidelines suggested in this chapter. When necessary, use the supplemental treatment strategies presented in chapter 6 to help you achieve your goals and lead a more fulfilling lifestyle. Continue to assess for progressive changes in your mood. As you are experimenting with your behaviors, continue to ask yourself whether your behavioral changes are resulting in increased feelings of reward or accomplishment. Are feelings of sadness, depression, and anxiety decreasing at all? Also, always remember to modify your weekly assignments based on the progress you are making in treatment. Good progress means you should continue to move forward with activating different behaviors. Slow progress means you should think about why it is difficult to complete your behaviors. Are there obstacles preventing you from completing your goals? Are you setting unrealistic expectations for yourself? Do you need to learn the additional skills presented in chapter 6? Do you need to revisit your Life-Goal Assessment and determine if you forgot about or ignored important life areas that should be included in your treatment? Try to be a good observer of your behavior. Learn about yourself, what is important to you, and how you can continue to change the way you behave to lead a more satisfying life.

RUMINATION-CUED ACTIVATION

Rumination refers to very negative and continuous thinking patterns, or chronic worrying. As a second goal over these next several weeks, we would like you build upon your behavioral activation skills by learning another skill called rumination-cued activation (Addis and Martell 2001). *Rumination-cued activation* refers to the process of learning how to activate your behaviors when rumination occurs, which also can be thought of as having intrusive or worrisome thoughts related to your depression and anxiety. In behavior therapy, the emphasis is on changing behaviors and experiences to bring about positive changes in thoughts, mood, and life satisfaction. However, we also recognize that there will be times when you will have depressive or anxious thoughts and that sometimes these thoughts will be fairly frequent, intense, and negative. In these cases you may not know what to do. When you encounter a difficult situation, it is completely natural to experience negative emotions or negative thoughts for a period of time. Often, these negative emotions and thoughts will be useful in terms of helping you resolve situations or problems. However, there comes a time when thinking (or ruminating) excessively is counterproductive and prevents you from engaging in particular behaviors or activities. As other psychologists have explained (Addis and Martell 2001), you know you're ruminating if:

> You're thinking over and over about negative thoughts, feelings, or situations (for example, persistently worrying about having cancer, being treated for cancer, side effects of treatment, issues of mortality, or how your cancer is affecting important people in your life).

> The process of thinking over and over again is not helping you feel less depressed, more hopeful, or less self-critical.

> The process of thinking has not helped you solve a problem.

So when you notice that you're ruminating, here's what you should do. First, use the rumination as a cue to *activate*. When you notice you are worrying excessively, engage in behaviors (in your hierarchy) that require attention or focus and thus are incompatible with rumination. Whether you decide to engage in an easier or more difficult behavior is up to you. The important point is that you engage in a behavior that will allow you to refocus your attention and thus prevent the urge to indulge and become highly preoccupied with your ruminations, a tendency that will not serve to improve your mood or accomplish life goals. Second, as you will learn later in this workbook, other strategies such as relaxation, mindfulness, and self-hypnosis may be included in your behavioral hierarchy to counteract the tendency to ruminate. Third, learn how to self-soothe through your five senses. Focus intensely on sights, sounds, scents, tastes, and touch. Appreciate and understand the world around you. Sit back and relax and take several deep breaths. Then, carefully think about and describe to yourself everything you see, hear, smell, and feel (in great detail). For example, if you are ruminating excessively about having cancer, work toward shifting the focus from cancer-related thoughts to what is going on in the present. Where are you currently? What kind of clothes are you wearing? Who is around you? What are they saying or doing? Can you hear anything? What does it sound like? What do you see? Are there any pleasurable or unusual fragrances in the air? Do you feel any sensations in your body?

EXERCISE: PRACTICE RUMINATION-CUED ACTIVATION

Think about something that you have been stressed about, something you have been ruminating about. Allow yourself to experience the worrisome thoughts. Once you have these thoughts clearly in your mind, let them go. Free your mind and focus on the world around you, all you see, hear, smell, and feel. Live in the present. Try to maintain your focus on your senses for approximately five minutes. If you find yourself suddenly distracted by ruminations, this is a signal to turn your focus back to what is happening in your world. When you are done, write about what your experience was like.

How did this experience relate to having negative thoughts? Did you have any intrusive thoughts while completing the exercise? How might this exercise be incorporated into your daily life? When are the times (days, hours, or situations) when you are most likely to ruminate? Can you schedule activities at these times to minimize the likelihood of ruminative experiences? Try to engage in rumination-cued activation whenever worrisome thoughts become too difficult to tolerate.

CONTINUE TO CONFRONT CANCER THROUGH BEHAVIORAL EXPOSURE

The last goal for this week (and the last cancer exposure exercise in this workbook) is to complete your work toward confronting your experience of living with cancer. Here is a final brief exposure assignment.

EXERCISE: LETTER TO MY FRIEND DIAGNOSED WITH CANCER

Please write a letter to one of your close friends whom you have just found out has been diagnosed with cancer (real or imagined). Try to be encouraging and supportive of your friend, and try to address common negative feelings, emotions, and thoughts that your friend might be experiencing. How would you recommend coping or thinking about the situation that might make it a little less difficult for him or her to handle? It might be helpful to touch on specific thoughts, fears, and emotional reactions that you experienced or continue to experience and how you deal with these issues. Again, there is no requirement for length. Just write as much as you need to fully describe this experience.

What was it like to write this letter? What did you learn about yourself? What did the exercise teach you about your ability to cope with cancer and to provide support to your friends? What emotions did you experience? Were they unwanted? Were they unwanted but in some way helpful, healing, or therapeutic? How was it different from trying to avoid the thoughts or experiences associated with living with cancer?

Congratulations for all the hard work you have put into activating your behavior. You are well on your way to overcoming your depression and anxiety and on the path to a healthier and more fulfilling lifestyle. As you continue on this journey, the remainder of this workbook is dedicated to providing you with supplementary behavioral activation skills and tools that may be worked into your Master Activity Log and Behavior Checkout—tools that will further assist you in overcoming your depression and anxiety.

CHAPTER 6

Treatment and Medication Management

Now that you are engaging in the behavioral activation component of the workbook and you have begun to expose yourself to some of the fear and anxiety that may have been related to being diagnosed and living with cancer, it's time to think about other factors that may be affecting your mood in a negative way or that might be contributing to an inability to effectively experience pleasure in your world. For example, sometimes the medical treatment you're receiving or the medications you are taking can cause side effects that affect your mood and your ability to enjoy life. Sometimes you may come across problems that might be difficult to solve that may also increase feelings of sadness and anxiety. Because of pain, depression, or anxiety, your sleep may be unsatisfying and you may be unable to relax. You may be finding it difficult to experience pleasure in social situations because you're anxious or feel unable to say or do the "right" things. As you continue to work toward improving your life through behavioral activation, the purpose of these next few chapters is to further assist you in dealing with these other important issues and to help you continue on the path toward a better quality of life.

MANAGING YOUR TREATMENT AND MEDICATION

Treatment noncompliance refers to the inability of a patient to keep scheduled appointments, refusal or inability to stick to recommended treatments, failure to report side effects of treatment, or an unwillingness to engage in supplemental treatment strategies such as those designed to treat depression or anxiety that might be related to cancer. Complying with cancer treatment is critical toward not only improving your physical health but also decreasing symptoms of depression and anxiety. A healthier body results in healthier psychological functioning, or a better ability to think rationally, behave with more energy and enthusiasm, and accomplish the goals that you've set for yourself. Even though the importance of complying with your cancer treatment should be clear, it's astounding how many cancer patients actually do not comply with treatment.

Several studies have demonstrated that many people with cancer are not adequately compliant with treatment. For example, one study found that approximately 23 percent of patients did not keep their appointments to receive chemotherapy (Itano et al. 1983). About 30 percent of women who had abnormal Pap smears and required follow-up care did not keep their appointments (Marcus et al. 1992). In an interesting study that was done with women diagnosed with breast cancer for at least two years who were receiving chemotherapy or hormone treatment, an amazing 46 percent said that they forgot to take their drugs and about 10 percent admitted they had intentionally decided not to take their medication (Atkins and Fallowfield 2006). Given that it's obvious that treatment compliance is essential for optimal medical and psychological health and the fact that many cancer patients do not comply with treatment, it's important to highlight reasons for treatment noncompliance and to discuss strategies useful for improving your ability to effectively engage in your treatment.

Reasons for Treatment Noncompliance and Potential Solutions

People who don't have cancer probably would have a very difficult time imagining the level of stress and difficulties involved in working through a cancer diagnosis. As we've addressed earlier in this workbook, having cancer often involves very complex emotional experiences that range from anxiety and depression, to confusion and anger, to pain and sickness. Often interspersed among these negative experiences are times of hope, optimism, and courage. It is difficult to imagine why cancer patients might refuse medications that might help them feel better and maybe even save their lives. We now know that noncompliance is really caused by many factors. We also know that being noncompliant with treatment doesn't necessarily mean a person is just being difficult. Indeed, amidst the stress and worries associated with cancer, being compliant with treatment can be extremely difficult, even for the most focused and committed of people.

INADEQUATE KNOWLEDGE ABOUT TREATMENT

Miscommunication or lack of information about cancer treatment may be a significant reason for noncompliance. For those of you who have already been involved in cancer treatment or are preparing for treatment, you know that cancer treatment may be complicated and involve many different steps. For example, following a surgical procedure to remove a malignant tumor, time-consuming and physically as well as emotionally draining radiation and chemotherapy interventions may be needed. Additional interventions to address psychological problems, nutritional issues, and other quality-of-life concerns may be necessary. If all treatment options are not properly explained and a clear plan is not outlined, cancer patients may not fully understand the importance of each treatment strategy and may decide not to pursue or to inadequately follow treatment recommendations.

Solution. Being more compliant with treatment will involve being ready to learn. Plan on being very active toward engaging in your treatment. Communication must be established early on in treatment and should involve open and thorough discussions with your primary care physician, oncologist, nurse, therapist, and family members. If you don't feel you're being heard or feel that people are not providing you with enough time to express your concerns and needs, be assertive about your thoughts and feelings (strategies are presented later in this chapter to help you with this process). Also, be prepared to ask lots of questions about your cancer diagnosis and treatment recommendations. If you find it hard to recall these questions, write them down before appointments. Also, seek out information through reading about cancer and perhaps surfing the Internet if access is available. Just as being educated about depression and anxiety is the first step toward overcoming these problems, educating yourself about cancer treatment is critical toward making sure you can follow your treatment appropriately. Finally, when meeting with your medical provider, take a small notebook along. Appointments happen very quickly, and usually a lot of information is provided in a brief period of time. Write down treatment recommendations, important dates, and other things to remember, such as whom to contact for follow-up psychological care, case management, or other treatment needs.

DEPRESSION AND ANXIETY

We designed this workbook because depression and anxiety can be overwhelming emotions. These emotional experiences can be so debilitating that they can prevent you from following through with prescribed treatments and can affect your ability to remember important information. In addition to affecting treatment compliance, these emotions, left untreated, can worsen your prognosis and even decrease your immunity to other medical problems.

Solution. As highlighted in the introduction, there are a number of treatment alternatives that are useful in helping you overcome depression and anxiety. These include using workbooks such as this one, becoming involved in individual or group psychotherapy, joining a support group, meeting with your psychiatrist or primary care physician to discuss the possibilities of psychotropic medications, or, after consulting with your medical provider, possibly incorporating an herbal treatment to assist you with emotional problems. Explore and think about these options, recognize the importance of treating depression and anxiety to improve compliance with cancer treatment, choose a plan, implement it, and evaluate its effectiveness.

BEING BUSY, FORGETFULNESS, AND LOGISTICAL ISSUES

There is no doubt that we live in a high-pressure society where we have many responsibilities. The more obligations we have, the easier it is to become overwhelmed and forget even the most important things. When you factor in the time associated with being diagnosed with and treated for cancer, this situation is made even more difficult. For example, taking time off of work, trying to arrange childcare, finding transportation, and putting all sorts of time into radiation therapy, chemotherapy, visits to the oncologist, going to the pharmacy, and contacting insurance companies and dealing with financial issues can require tremendous time commitments. When too many things are going on in your life, something has to give, and sometimes this is your commitment to following through with your cancer treatment.

Solution. It would be ideal if other people could take on some of the demanding responsibilities in your life. To some extent, maybe this is possible. Think about the resources you have, the people in your life who might be willing to make some sacrifices to assist you in your time of need. Don't be afraid to ask for help. All of us need assistance at certain points in our lives, and being diagnosed with and treated for cancer usually creates situations where help is going to be needed. Be an active problem solver and learn to proactively arrange your time and resources so as not to become completely overwhelmed (we'll discuss this further later in this chapter). Time-management skills are of the utmost importance. In addition to keeping a weekly planner or a detailed calendar, there are a variety of medication reminder systems that might be useful. These techniques can include the use of pill dispensers and organizers, vibrating alarm watches, alarm clocks, and beepers. More high-tech strategies such as personal digital assistants also could be useful in keeping track of your appointments, medications, and other pressing responsibilities. To further assist you in complying with treatment, keeping in close contact with someone who has had similar experiences, such as an acquaintance diagnosed with cancer, also may substantially improve your likelihood of feeling less overwhelmed and more likely to adhere to treatment.

MEANS OF EXERTING CONTROL

Being diagnosed with cancer may be associated with the experience of losing control of your life. Sudden changes happen whereby you can become overwhelmed by the additional time demands mentioned above, difficult experiences with pain and fatigue, and even increased financial burdens. This perceived lack of control can become overpowering, contribute to feelings of depression and anxiety, and cause a person to strive toward increased control. One of the less adaptive ways to regain some of this control can be to refuse to engage in some aspects of your cancer intervention. Although the consequences of such actions can be extreme and even life threatening, for some people with cancer, it is the only way they know how to take charge of their life.

Solution. The solution here is a simple one. Consistent with the earlier discussion on acceptance versus change (see chapter 5), there are some situations where people can actively work toward changing their situation and other circumstances where the best alternative is to accept difficult conditions and realize that they are only temporary. In the case of experiencing a lack of control, this is a normal response to all that you are experiencing in living a life with cancer. The best way to cope with these feelings of being out of control is through gaining a sense of power over your disease, an outcome that will occur in the course of sticking with your treatment plan and successfully overcoming your illness. So we ask that you be aware of these control issues in your life and be sure to prevent issues of control from negatively impacting your treatment compliance. Remember that your participation in the behavioral activation component of this workbook is a much more acceptable and helpful method to control your life and your time.

DIFFICULTY SWALLOWING PILLS

A significant number of people have a problem with swallowing pills. The anxiety associated with swallowing pills can be overwhelming, especially when one anticipates that certain medications can cause unwanted side effects. Tastes of certain medications also can be highly unappealing, which may further contribute to noncompliance.

Solution. People have been quite creative in their efforts to overcome fears around swallowing pills. Crushing or splitting pills may be effective, while other people choose to mix their pills with food, perhaps something like yogurt or applesauce. More recently, there also are a couple of products that are available to assist with this problem. Low-cost sprays are available to coat pills with a more appealing taste, and specially designed pill-swallowing cups also may provide some relief from this problem.

SIDE EFFECTS OF MEDICATIONS

Many people with cancer skip appointments or refuse medications because of a fear of side effects such as nausea, fatigue, hair loss, and vomiting. Side effects will in part depend on the type of drug, dosage, other medications you are taking, the time of day you're taking the drug, and how long you've been on the medication. Although it is true that for many people substantial side effects do not necessarily occur with treatment, for others these are difficult consequences to endure as part of cancer treatment.

Solution. There are a number of strategies to minimize the likelihood that fears about side effects will limit your compliance with cancer treatment. First, it will help if you become educated about the treatment you are receiving and learn what to expect. Second, you can make some dietary changes that will allow you to control some symptoms such as nausea and vomiting. This might include eating smaller meals as well as foods that are not overly spicy, fatty, or salty. Third, to the extent possible, engage in some mild to moderate exercise. This will help to strengthen your body and immune system to cope with the medications you are taking. Fourth, learn strategies such as those outlined in this workbook to control your anxiety and depression. The more anxious or depressed you are, the more difficult it will be to tolerate medications. Fifth, there are a number of medications that you can ask for that will help to control symptoms such as nausea and vomiting. Ask your doctor if these might be useful for you. Sixth, you may decide to cope with a side effect in a more proactive way. For example, if you are likely to lose your hair from a certain medication, you may decide to cut it off before it falls out. Many cancer survivors highly endorse this strategy and suggest it was probably easier than slowly watching hair loss. Seventh, if you are feeling considerable fatigue, remember that this is normal and it is okay to feel this way. Do not overwork yourself, and utilize friends and family members to assist you with responsibilities.

Eighth, if you experience mouth soreness as a result of using some chemotherapy drugs, consider a less spicy diet and avoid fruit juices for a while. Finally, and most importantly, remember that these side effects are only temporary. Take care of your illness, comply with your treatment, work through the side effects, and in time you will once again have your life back.

EXERCISE: IMPROVING TREATMENT COMPLIANCE

As you read through the previous section, what issues seemed most likely to limit your ability to comply with your cancer treatment?

_____

_____

_____

_____

_____

What is your plan for dealing with these issues so that you can successfully engage in treatment?

_____

_____

_____

_____

_____

_____

Now that you have learned the importance of being compliant with your treatment, we hope that you will follow physician and oncologist recommendations as they are given to you. We also hope that your compliance with medical treatment generalizes to being compliant with the exercises proposed to you in this workbook. Indeed, we would like you to consider the behavioral exercises in the same way you would think about receiving medications or another form of treatment. The exercises in this workbook are in essence a prescription—a prescription for improved mental health. As you work through the next several chapters, continue your hard work and remember that you are learning skills that will remain with you for a long time and will assist you in becoming a healthier, more fulfilled person.

CHAPTER 7

Becoming an Effective Problem Solver

TIME: Approximately One Week

There is a good body of research that speaks to the fact that cancer patients often report increased problems and daily hassles as a result of being diagnosed with and living with cancer (Newell, Sanson-Fisher, and Savolamin 2002; Nezu et al. 1999). These problems may involve many different aspects of your life, including logistical problems, financial stress, disruptions within your social system, increased conflict with friends and family, changing responsibilities, increased drug and alcohol use, or decreased engagement in behaviors, activities, or hobbies that you used to find enjoyable. To be certain, all of us have problems that creep into our lives, but a significant life stressor such as having cancer can compound these problems.

Thankfully, some major progress has been made toward developing a systematic approach to helping cancer patients resolve problems more effectively—approaches shared in this section (Mynors-Wallis 2005; Nezu 1989; Nezu et al. 1999; Stanley, Diefenbach, and Hopko 2004). The purpose of this part of the workbook is to provide another skill for you to use. More specifically, the goal is to allow you to learn how to build upon your behavioral activation skills by teaching you to more efficiently solve problems that you may experience in your life.

PROBLEM-SOLVING TREATMENT RATIONALE

Problem-solving treatment is based upon the idea that your symptoms of anxiety and depression are often caused by practical problems you face in everyday life. The goal is to offer you a clearer structure within which you can better resolve your problems, with the expectation that your depression and anxiety symptoms will improve as your problems resolve. Problem-solving treatment is very much in the present, or "here and now." In other words, the treatment focuses on your current difficulties and helps to establish goals for the future. The treatment does not dwell on past relationships and past mistakes, but instead focuses on what you can more actively work toward changing—namely, the present.

The Goals of Problem Solving

All of us have problems, some of which are more difficult to solve than others. Unresolved problems in our lives can cause us to feel down or blue. They can make us feel like our life is getting out of control and is overwhelming us. *Problem-solving treatment* is a structured approach for learning to clarify your problems and find useful solutions for them. As you start to make progress toward solving your problems more effectively, you'll find that you will begin to feel more in control of your life, and with this increased feeling of control, you will experience less depression and anxiety. Remember that improvement is most likely to occur following action, so we put a lot of emphasis on providing you with important problem-solving tasks that will help you build these skills.

With problem-solving treatment, there are four major goals (Mynors-Wallis 2005). The first goal is to increase your understanding of the connection between your current symptoms and everyday problems. With this, it needs to be understood that problems are a part of everyday life, and effectively resolving these problems will in turn improve how you are feeling. The second goal of problem-solving treatment is to increase your ability to clearly and accurately define your current problems. What we really want to teach is the importance of setting concrete and realistic goals for problem solving. Third, we want to teach you a specific problem-solving method in an attempt to help you solve your problems in a structured manner. This is where we will introduce problem-solving skills and practice these skills using real-life problems that you are currently trying to resolve. The last goal of this problem-solving treatment is to produce a greater number of positive experiences as a result of your ability to solve problems. This will increase your confidence when it comes to solving future problems and also increase your feelings of self-control during problematic situations. Through achieving all four of these goals you will be able to better cope with problems in the future and thus avoid or minimize further emotional distress.

DESIGNING A PROBLEM-SOLVING LIST

The first goal of problem-solving treatment is to make a list of your current problems. Now that you are aware of how problems may be strongly associated with symptoms of depression and anxiety, it's time to begin to use problem solving to more effectively deal with your life and assist you in starting to feel better. Obviously, in order for you to learn to better solve your problems, we need to get a sense of what sorts of problems you are currently experiencing and decide on where to begin. So let's take some time to learn about some specific things that might be bothering you right now. As you think about what these problems might be, for now focus on the broad picture of your problems. In other words, you will get more specific about your problems as you work through the remainder of this section. For now, as you develop the problem-solving list below, focus on generally describing your problems within each of the areas specified. These problems can be minor and major, coming from all areas of your life.

EXERCISE: MY PROBLEM LIST

Under the following life areas, write down problems you might be experiencing.

RELATIONSHIP WITH PARTNER/SPOUSE: _____

_____

_____

RELATIONSHIPS WITH CHILDREN, PARENTS, SIBLINGS, AND OTHER FAMILY MEMBERS: ____

_____

_____

RELATIONSHIPS WITH FRIENDS: _____

_____

_____

ENGAGING IN BEHAVIORS, ACTIVITIES, OR HOBBIES YOU FIND ENJOYABLE: _____

_____

_____

SPIRITUALITY: _____

_____

_____

WORK: _____

_____

MONEY: _____

_____

_____

HOUSING: _____

_____

_____

HEALTH: _____

_____

_____

LEGAL ISSUES: _____

_____

_____

ALCOHOL AND DRUGS: _____

_____

_____

OTHER: _____

_____

_____

PROBLEM SOLVED

Now that you have created your problem list, think about how these problems might be contributing to your depression and anxiety. Think about the difficulties you are having, how many problems you identified, how often these problems are occurring, and how they may increase feelings of anxiety and depression. Remember that these symptoms are largely a response to your problems. If problems are not being effectively solved, or even avoided (recall chapter 4), you can expect that symptoms of anxiety and depression will continue to persist. So in the interest of feeling less anxious and depressed, let's begin the process of becoming a better problem solver. Remember, it's important that you play an active role in learning how to problem solve. Over time, as you practice the process of problem solving, it will become more natural for you. For now, however, you will learn to be an effective problem solver by following very specific steps through use of a process called "SOLVED."

S = Selecting a Problem

The first step in problem solving is to evaluate the situation that creates depression and anxiety and to select a specific problem to be solved. It's important to be specific and try to evaluate realistically whether the problem identified is reasonable and solvable. For this first exercise, it would be best to tackle one of the smaller problems on your problem list, but one that is significant to you all the same. It's not absolutely crucial which specific problem you choose for this exercise, but it's important to choose a problem that you feel you can make some progress on rather than choosing one that is going to overwhelm you. So for now, let's not try to work through solving the problem of world hunger or ending terrorism. Let's focus on a simpler problem that you have been experiencing recently. As you gain more experience at problem solving, you can tackle more difficult problems.

Using the sample SOLVED Worksheet provided as an example, use the SOLVED Worksheet #1 to write down your specific problem (SOLVED Worksheet #2 should be photocopied multiple times for later use). In clarifying your problem, it would be best for you to ask yourself these four questions and summarize your responses under "S" on your worksheet:

1. What is the problem?

2. When does the problem occur?

3. Where does the problem occur?

4. Who is involved in the problem?

O = Open Your Mind to All Possible Solutions

The second stage of the problem-solving process involves identifying as many possible solutions to the problem as you can think of. Here, it is important to be as broad as possible. We would like you to do what is called *brainstorming*, which refers to writing down every possible solution that comes to mind, without consideration of the consequences. Be creative and write down anything that comes to mind on SOLVED Worksheet #1. The greater the number of possible solutions, the greater the chances that you will successfully resolve your problem. Remember that the first idea that comes to mind is not always the best idea. Also, feel free to combine your ideas and modify them as you think about them further. Don't worry about judging your ideas until the brainstorming process is complete. Prematurely judging could cost you a potentially successful solution. If you are having problems thinking of solutions, try to think about how other people would act in your shoes. Think about what advice you would give someone else with this problem. Look at the ways that you and others might handle similar situations. You may even wish to consult with a close friend or family member who you think might be able to offer potential solutions. Potentials solutions should not be discarded or prejudged, even if initially they seem to be silly or unworkable. Remember that the goal here is to help you think of multiple solutions so you can become more flexible in solving your problems. In order to facilitate your brainstorming, it can be helpful to make the following statements to yourself: "What else can you think of?" "Think freely," "Be playful with your ideas," "Don't prejudge or evaluate your ideas right now."

Another way to think about the brainstorming process is to deliberately invent a solution that is absolutely silly. Just remember to think freely and be creative when you brainstorm, and solutions will come to you in no time. Remember that you are the expert in your life and are much more likely than anyone else to be aware of your circumstances and come up with relevant and workable solutions to your problems. After you have generated as many potential solutions as possible to your problem, the next step will be to choose a solution that you will implement.

L = List the Costs and Benefits

Now that you have identified multiple solutions to your problem, the next step is to evaluate and choose one or more of these solutions to implement. As presented in the sample SOLVED Worksheet, this step involves examining all of the advantages (benefits or pros) and disadvantages (costs or cons) of putting each of the solutions into action. Try to think about how each solution will impact your problem, and write down the costs and benefits on SOLVED Worksheet #1. How will each solution be useful, and how could it be less useful or even harmful toward solving your problem? How will this solution affect your time, effort, money, and emotional situation? What positive and negative effects might this solution have on your friends and family? Do you see yourself being able to carry out this plan of action in a satisfactory manner?

V = Verify the Best Solution and Create a Plan

Now that you have looked more closely at your potential solutions, how do you think they compare? Considering all of them, which solution has the most benefits associated with it and the least cost? Which solution do you think is the best for your problem? Do you see this solution as one that shows a high likelihood of you achieving your goal and overcoming your problem? In some situations, remember that the easiest solution is not always the best solution. For example, in the sample SOLVED Worksheet, the easiest solution might have been to stop driving completely. However, when reviewing the costs and benefits associated with this course of action, you can see that not driving would have resulted in too many costs or restrictions on this person's life. So remember that you want to choose a doable solution that might involve more effort but also might allow you to have a better balance of increased benefits and fewer costs.

Once you have carefully assessed the benefits and costs associated with each potential solution, rank order these solutions on SOLVED Worksheet #1, with 1 being the most preferred solution and 5 being the least preferred solution. Remember that, ideally, the most preferred solution selected should achieve your goals and also have the least personal and interpersonal disadvantages associated with it. After you have identified the most preferred solution, create a plan for carrying it out. Identify the steps needed to carry out your plan. For example, In the sample SOLVED Worksheet, this person had the most preferred solution of "learning to overcome my anxiety about driving." For this person, learning to overcome her anxiety involved a plan of developing better coping skills to use when she was driving. First, she learned how to better relax to manage her anxiety (using the progressive muscle-relaxation strategy presented in a later chapter). Being more relaxed allowed her to feel more at ease when behind the wheel. Second, with the help of a therapist, she developed a plan to learn to gradually expose herself to driving while using her relaxation skills. The plan involved having her progress from simply sitting in her car (not started) in her driveway, to sitting in her driveway with the car started, to driving around the block with her husband in the car, to driving around the block by herself, to driving to the grocery store with her husband, to driving to the grocery store without her husband, and so forth.

E = Enact the Plan

In the fifth stage of problem solving, you carry out the plan outlined in the previous step. Now that you have chosen a solution and tentative plan of the most appropriate way to achieve your goals, firm up your plan of action by being as detailed as possible. Think about dates, times, places, and people who will be involved in carrying out your plan. If the situation dictates, you can even get as detailed as planning what you're going to say. Make sure you are clear about what needs to be done, where it will happen, whom it involves, and how it will be done. Make sure you have chosen a plan that you will feel comfortable implementing. If you are anxious about carrying out a plan, decide how you will cope with that anxiety. You might want to learn how to better relax or might want to role play with other people to practice what you will say or do. If you are ruminating or worrying excessively, remember the rumination-cued activation you learned in chapter 5. Your worry is a sign that you must take action and work toward solving an issue.

D = Decide If Your Solution Worked

In the final stage of problem-solving treatment, the evaluation phase, you need to ask yourself whether the selected solution and plan that were implemented were effective. Were the solution and plan effective in resolving the problem you outlined in the first stage of this treatment? If so, congratulate yourself for a job well done and recognize the progress you have made toward becoming a more effective problem solver. How did effectively solving the problem impact your feeling of depression and anxiety? Did solving the problem help with these emotions? Remember the link between life problems and anxiety and depressive symptoms. Even if you did not sense an immediate change in your mood after effectively solving your problem, be patient and persistent. Change sometimes takes time.

In some cases your plan may not have been effective toward solving your problem. Be careful not to become too discouraged if this happens. Try to avoid falling into the trap of becoming overly focused on "failing," as many people with depression and anxiety are prone to do. Instead, examine the possible reasons for the difficulties you're having. Consider if the problem and goals should be defined more clearly. Were the goals realistic? Was the plan realistic? Did any new obstacles arise that might have prevented you from resolving the problem? How can these be dealt with effectively? Were the implementation steps difficult to achieve? If so, why? If the plan was enacted successfully and did not result in solving the problem, think about whether an alternative solution listed in "O" might be more effective. If you didn't experience benefits in your mood after solving your problem, remember that depression and anxiety symptoms often develop over weeks to months and it is unlikely that they will resolve immediately. When someone goes on a diet, they can't expect to lose all the weight in the first week. Like using behavioral activation, change using problem-solving treatment will take time. Be patient, practice, and you will find a problem-solving strategy to help you be less depressed and anxious and a more effective person in this world.

SAMPLE SOLVED WORKSHEET

1. **S**ELECT THE PROBLEM

I am anxious about driving my car. Happens all the time, when going anywhere.

2. **O**PEN YOUR MIND TO ALL POSSIBLE SOLUTIONS

    A. *Stop driving completely.*

    B. *Have someone else drive me places.*

    C. *Take public transportation.*

    D. *Learn to overcome my anxiety about driving.*

    E. *Walk instead of driving.*

3. **L**IST THE COSTS OF EACH SOLUTION

    A. *Very restricted in what I can do, more anxiety and depression.*

    B. *Burdensome for others, don't get over anxiety.*

    C. *Be with strangers, maybe dangerous, takes longer to travel.*

    D. *Might initially involve increased anxiety, time and money for therapy.*

    E. *Places too far to walk, too hard on my body.*

BENEFITS

A. *No more anxiety.*

B. *No more anxiety, company, can get things done.*

C. *No more anxiety, get things done, won't have to do car maintenance.*

D. *Can have more flexibility, drive myself, don't have to rely on others.*

E. *Exercise, cheap.*

4. **V**ERIFY THE BEST SOLUTION (RANK ORDER: 1 = best, 5 = worst)

A. *4*

B. *3*

C. *2*

D. *1*

E. *5*

5. **E**NACT YOUR PLAN

6. **D**ECIDE IF YOUR SOLUTION WORKED   (YES)   NO

SOLVED WORKSHEET #1

1. **S**ELECT THE PROBLEM

2. **O**PEN YOUR MIND TO ALL POSSIBLE SOLUTIONS

    A. _____

    B. _____

    C. _____

    D. _____

    E. _____

3. **L**IST THE COSTS OF EACH SOLUTION

    A. _____

    B. _____

    C. _____

    D. _____

    E. _____

    BENEFITS

    A. _____

    B. _____

    C. _____

    D. _____

    E. _____

4. **V**ERIFY THE BEST SOLUTION (RANK ORDER)

    A. _____

    B. _____

    C. _____

    D. _____

    E. _____

5. **E**NACT YOUR PLAN

6. **D**ECIDE IF YOUR SOLUTION WORKED   YES   NO

SOLVED WORKSHEET #2

1. **S**ELECT THE PROBLEM

2. **O**PEN YOUR MIND TO ALL POSSIBLE SOLUTIONS

   A. _____

   B. _____

   C. _____

   D. _____

   E. _____

3. **L**IST THE COSTS OF EACH SOLUTION

   A. _____

   B. _____

   C. _____

   D. _____

   E. _____

   BENEFITS

   A. _____

   B. _____

   C. _____

   D. _____

   E. _____

4. **V**ERIFY THE BEST SOLUTION (RANK ORDER)

   A. _____

   B. _____

   C. _____

   D. _____

   E. _____

5. **E**NACT YOUR PLAN

6. **D**ECIDE IF YOUR SOLUTION WORKED   YES   NO

An inability to solve problems effectively has been shown to greatly increase stress and the subsequent development of depression and anxiety problems. The problem-solving skills you have learned in this chapter will go a long way toward providing you with an additional strategy to overcome difficult situations and reduce problems with your emotions. This is one of several key strategies that will help with your emotions, with others presented in the remainder of this workbook. We now move toward discussing another problem that may be related to depression and anxiety: getting an inadequate or unfulfilling night's sleep.

CHAPTER 8

Getting a More Restful Night's Sleep

TIME: Approximately One Week

It is a well-known fact that people with cancer often do not get as restful a sleep as people who do not have cancer (Akechi et al. 2006; Berger, Sankaranarayanan, and Watanabe-Galloway 2006; Fernandes et al. 2006). Compared to healthy people, cancer patients report being more fatigued, having worse sleep quality, lower daytime activity levels, and worse quality of life (Fernandes et al. 2006). Adults with cancer also seem to be particularly prone to developing problems that affect the normal cycle of sleeping and waking. These problems can involve difficulties getting up in the morning, waking up during the night, and daytime sleepiness. In fact, most adults with cancer wake up several times during the night, and it has been suggested that almost 50 percent of cancer patients may experience a sleep disorder, with insomnia being the most common (Lee et al. 2004; Theobald 2004).

NORMAL SLEEP

Sleep is necessary for everyone's health and well-being. When people are not sleeping well, their immune functions or ability to fight off illness may be compromised. Poor sleep also can affect the way you handle stressful experiences and impact your daytime activities and quality of life (Lee et al. 2004). The process of sleep involves fairly predictable cycles that occur at approximately ninety-minute intervals throughout the course of the night. You have about five or six cycles in a normal night's sleep that consists of about eight hours. These cycles generally begin by entering what is referred to as *non–rapid eye movement* (NREM) sleep. NREM sleep consists of four different stages that range from very light sleep (stage 1 or alpha wave sleep) to very deep sleep or delta wave sleep (stage 4). So, as you become drowsy at night, you will enter stage I sleep, progress through stage 4 sleep, then return to stage I sleep, at which point rapid eye movement (REM) sleep will begin. It is during this REM sleep that most of your dream life occurs. Over the course of a night's sleep, you will have approximately five or six REM episodes, with the length of these episodes increasing as the night progresses.

Human beings also experience what is referred to as circadian patterns or circadian rhythms. *Circadian rhythms* involve your body's biological clock, or the tendency to engage in sleep behavior at certain times during the day. A part of your brain called the *hypothalamus* is strongly related to these circadian rhythms and helps you to know when it's time to go to sleep. Circadian rhythms are affected by many factors that may include your social interactions, when you eat, and when you work but, most importantly, the cycle of light and darkness. Because many of these factors differ across people, along with other circumstances (for instance, level of sleep deprivation, physical fitness, other behavioral patterns), circadian-rhythm patterns may differ, with some people preferring early bedtimes and wake times and others preferring later bedtimes and wake times.

WHAT IS INSOMNIA?

The prevalence of insomnia is higher among women and older persons, but it generally seems to occur in about 30 percent of the population (National Sleep Foundation 2007). Sleep disturbance, or *insomnia*, can include difficulty falling asleep (taking more than thirty minutes), problems maintaining sleep (waking more than twice during the night), and awakening too early from a night's sleep. As a result of these difficulties, a number of problems can occur during the day, including daytime sleepiness, fatigue, mood problems, social problems, and attention or memory impairment. It is important to remember that not all people require the same amount of sleep at night. Although about 65 percent of adults require about seven to eight hours of sleep per night, the remaining one-third of adults may be either short sleepers (about four to five hours of sleep per night) or long sleepers (requiring about nine or ten hours of sleep). Interestingly, depending on factors such as the length of time it takes to fall asleep, frequency and duration of awakenings after falling asleep, and sleep efficiency, short sleepers may not have insomnia and long sleepers may still have insomnia (Morin 1993).

SLEEP PROBLEMS IN PEOPLE WITH CANCER

As indicated earlier, as many as 50 percent of cancer patients may have problems with insomnia. There is some evidence to suggest that problems with insomnia may increase substantially following a cancer diagnosis. For example, in a study of three hundred women diagnosed with breast cancer, although about 19 percent reported problems with insomnia prior to being diagnosed with cancer, after being diagnosed, 33 percent of the women indicated insomnia had become problematic (Savard et al. 2001). Although all cancer types may be associated with an increased likelihood of developing insomnia, it appears as though people with lung and breast cancer may be particularly likely to develop problems (Davidson et al. 2002). Given the fairly common occurrence of sleep problems among cancer patients, it is important to highlight the reasons why these sleep problems may occur.

Preexisting Factors

As we mentioned earlier, if you are an older person (over the age of sixty years) or female, you are at a slightly higher risk for already having sleep problems, even prior to a diagnosis of cancer. Indeed, regardless of your age or gender, you may already have been diagnosed with a common sleep disorder before being diagnosed with cancer, disorders that might include insomnia, sleep apnea, narcolepsy, or restless legs syndrome. Similarly, before being diagnosed with cancer, you may have had a number of lifestyle issues that may have been negatively affecting your sleep (Morin 1993). For example, several drugs may decrease the quantity and quality of sleep. These drugs might include caffeine, nicotine, alcohol, marijuana, and various amphetamines. Even prescription drugs may be partially related to insomnia. These drugs include various steroids, asthma medications (for instance, various bronchodilators), some beta blockers used to control hypertension (such as propranolol and clonidine), and even some antidepressant medications such as fluoxetine (Prozac).

In addition to drugs or medications, poor sleeping patterns may increase problems with insomnia. Such behaviors would include keeping irregular and unpredictable sleep patterns or schedules, excessive daytime napping, spending too much time in bed (even when awake), and using your bedroom for nonsleeping activities that might involve things like eating, watching television, or reading. Other patterns of behaving that might include poor nutrition and eating or exercising too soon before bedtime also could negatively affect your sleep. Obvious but sometimes overlooked factors that might hinder your sleep might involve too much noise or light in your bedroom, a room temperature that is too hot or too cold, and an uncomfortable mattress. Finally, certain negative attitudes and beliefs about sleep may be affecting your quality of sleep, such as putting too much pressure on yourself to sleep, having unrealistic sleep expectations, or overly focusing on and exaggerating the negative consequences of not falling asleep quickly. We'll address all of these issues in this chapter as we provide you with strategies to improve your sleep.

Cancer-Related Causes

Certain factors that are related to your cancer also may be affecting your sleep quality. For example, your sleep might be more affected if you have lung or breast cancer. The higher or more severe the stage of your cancer, the more likely it is that your sleep will be disrupted. Also, the more recently you have been through cancer treatment, or if you currently are going through cancer treatment, the more likely it is that you are having sleep difficulties (Davidson et al. 2002). Related to cancer treatment, certain side effects also may decrease sleep quality, including nausea, vomiting, diarrhea, or frequent need to urinate. Being in unfamiliar situations or environments such as hospitals also can cause significant sleep disturbance. A group of researchers recently reported that getting up earlier than usual to commute to morning treatment appointments may also be a precipitating factor toward insomnia (Lee et al. 2004). Finally, increases in pain predicted more difficulty getting to sleep and more problems waking up during the night (Palesh et al. 2006). Cancer-related pain is a significant problem that is believed to affect as many as 70 percent of cancer patients during the course of their illness. In one study that included over one thousand patients with metastatic cancer, 50 percent of the patients who reported cancer-related pain (about 70 percent of all cancer patients) indicated the pain was severe enough to impair their ability to perform their daily functions and responsibilities (Cleeland et al. 1994).

Stress, Anxiety, and Depression

In addition to pain, depression and anxiety have long been determined to negatively affect sleep (Barlow et al. 2002; Thase 2006). The relationship is a bidirectional one, however, and inadequate sleep can also increase depression and anxiety symptoms. Whatever the direction of causality between decreased sleep and emotions such as anxiety and depression, your quality of sleep can be greatly hindered if you are struggling emotionally. For example, higher levels of depression are associated with problems getting up in the morning, fewer hours of sleep, waking up during the night, and daytime sleepiness (Palesh et al. 2006). Greater life stress, social changes, family concerns, and financial stress among cancer patients also are linked with more problems getting to sleep and more daytime sleepiness (Palesh et al. 2006). These findings suggest that psychological distress is a possible key cause of sleep disturbance, and management of psychological distress may be one promising strategy for prevention of sleep disturbance among cancer patients (Akechi et al. 2006).

EXERCISE: FACTORS THAT MIGHT BE AFFECTING MY SLEEP

As you read through the above factors associated with sleep disturbance, which factors do you think might be limiting your ability to get a good night's sleep?

_____

_____

_____

_____

_____

STRATEGIES FOR OVERCOMING YOUR SLEEP PROBLEMS

Sleep difficulties are one of the most prominent concerns of cancer patients, and improving your sleep might help to reduce symptoms of depression, anxiety, and pain, and may even assist your immune system and ability to overcome cancer by increasing natural killer-cell activity (Irwin et al. 1995). Prior to learning very specific strategies for overcoming your sleep problems, it is useful to get a clearer picture of your sleep experiences. The process of learning more about how you currently sleep will help to better establish the severity of your sleep problem, may help you to connect problems with sleeping with certain behaviors and daily experiences that you have, and may also serve as a useful baseline with which you can monitor improvements in your sleep.

Keeping a Sleep Diary

With these goals in mind, the idea is that you will maintain a sleep diary over the next week (Morin 1993). When you awaken in the morning, you should answer all ten questions in your sleep diary. So, when you wake up on Thursday morning, complete the column under Thursday. When you awaken on Friday morning, complete the column under Friday, and so forth. Remember that it is important to do this every day and preferably as soon as possible after you awaken. This will help you to more accurately remember the information. It may be difficult to accurately and specifically recall some of the time periods that are being requested. We only ask that you do your very best to come up with as accurate a number as possible. The following guidelines will be helpful in answering the questions presented on the diary (Morin 1993):

> *Napping*: Include all naps, even if they were not intentional (for example, you fell asleep for fifteen minutes while your spouse was driving you to the doctor). Make sure to specify A.M. or P.M.

> *Sleep aid*: Include both prescribed and over-the-counter medications as well as alcohol used specifically as a sleep aid.

> *Bedtime*: This is when you actually go to bed and turn off the lights.

> *Sleep-onset latency*: Provide your best estimate of how long it took you to fall asleep after you turned off the lights.

> *Number of awakenings*: Record the number of times you remember waking up during the night.

> *Duration of awakenings*: Estimate to the best of your memory how many minutes you were awake each time you awoke during the night. Do not count your very last awakening that occurs in the morning.

Morning awakening: This is the last time you woke up in the morning. If you woke up at 5:30 A.M. and never went back to sleep, write 5:30. If you woke up at 5:30 A.M., were awake for one hour, and then fell asleep from 6:30 to 7:00 A.M., then your last awakening would be 7:00 A.M.

Out-of-bed time: This is the time you actually got out of your bed.

Feeling upon arising: 1 = Exhausted, 2 = Tired, 3 = Average, 4 = Refreshed, 5 = Very Refreshed

Sleep quality: 1 = Very Restless, 2 = Restless, 3 = Average, 4 = Sound, 5 = Very Sound

SLEEP DIARY

Date _____ to _____	Example	Mon	Tue	Wed	Thu	Fri	Sat	Sun
Yesterday, I napped from ____ to ____ (note the time of all naps).	12:00 to 1:30 P.M.							
Yesterday, I took ____ mg of medication and/or ____ oz of alcohol as a sleep aid.	Xanax .5 mg							
Last night, I went to bed and turned the lights off at ____ o'clock.	10:30							
After turning the lights out, I fell asleep in ____ minutes.	45 min							
My sleep was interrupted ____ times (specify number of nighttime awakenings).	2							
My sleep was interrupted for ____ minutes (specify duration of each awakening).	25, 35							
This morning, I woke up at ____ o'clock (note time of last awakening).	5:30							
This morning, I got out of bed at ____ o'clock (specify the time).	6:15							
When I got up this morning I felt ____. (1=Exhausted, 5=Refreshed)	2							
Overall, my sleep last night was ____. (1=Very Restless, 5=Very Sound).	2							

EXERCISE: WHAT I NOTICED ABOUT MY SLEEP PATTERN

Now that you have completed your weekly diary, there are several pieces of information that you should give close attention to. In particular, notice how many times per day (and for how long) you are napping. Look at how often you are using sleep aids. Roughly how long is it taking you to fall asleep? Is your sleep frequently interrupted? If so, can you identify any reasons? Do you usually wake up at the same time each morning? How do you feel in the morning? Was there anything you noticed that surprised you? What seems to be most problematic about your sleep?

_____

_____

_____

_____

_____

_____

_____

_____

Stimulus-Control Training

Now that you have a better idea of your sleep patterns and problems with achieving a good night's rest, it's time to focus on learning strategies to improve your sleep. There are two main behavioral strategies you can learn to improve the quality of your sleep: stimulus-control training and sleep hygiene (Perlis et al. 2004). We are asking that you learn these two strategies and try them out for a period of two weeks to see if your sleep improves.

Stimulus-control training refers to the idea that you have learned certain associations between your environment (in this case your bedroom) and behaviors (such as worrying, reading, and watching television) that are making it more difficult for you to sleep. Therefore, this treatment involves teaching you to make new associations to assist you in having a more restful sleep. In other words, the goal is to decrease the amount of time you spend awake in bed and eliminate behaviors that might be interfering with a good night's rest. To accomplish this goal, we ask that you learn the following rules and apply them over the next two weeks. Stick to these rules very carefully and consistently to see if they will be helpful to you, as they have been for many people we have treated in therapy. We use the acronym "SLEEP" as a shorthand for the steps you should take.

S = SET A REGULAR BEDTIME AND WAKE TIME

It is important for you to go to sleep at the same time every night and wake up at the same time every morning. Review your bedtimes and wake times as you noted in your sleep diary assignment. Are you going to bed and waking up at the same times? We encourage you to think about setting your bedtime at about 10:00 P.M. to 1:00 A.M. and to not expect to sleep for more than six to eight hours. Set your alarm clock so that you wake up at the same time every day, regardless of whether it is a weekday or weekend. Even if you didn't sleep well the previous night and might be tempted to sleep longer, do your best to stick with this routine. It will be important for regulating your internal biological clock. Actually, when you get used to it, getting up at a regular time can create new pleasures with some early morning activity (for instance, walking, reading the paper, or having some coffee) before the day begins. In addition to going to sleep at the same time, it will be most beneficial to you if you fall asleep fairly soon after lying down in bed. What you will do if you don't fall asleep within fifteen to twenty minutes will be covered below.

L = LIMIT THE USE OF YOUR BEDROOM

Limit the use of the bedroom to sleep or sex. It's important to associate the bedroom and bed only with behaviors that are productive for your sleep (or enjoyable) and to decrease the association between your bed and the experience of lying there, tossing and turning. So this means there are certain behaviors that you should no longer plan on doing in your bed. These include worrying, watching television, listening to the radio, reading, eating, and working. If you like to read to relax or listen to soft music to get sleepy for the evening, put on your pajamas and sit in a chair to read or listen to your music until you are sleepy enough to go to bed.

E = EXIT THE BEDROOM

When you go to bed at your regular time but then don't fall asleep within fifteen to twenty minutes, you should get up and go into another room until you feel sleepy. Again, this helps to increase the association of the bed and bedroom with sleeping, not hanging out awake and worrying about when you'll get to sleep. When you go into another room, feel free to engage in some quiet activity that might involve watching a movie (preferably one that doesn't induce strong emotional experiences), reading, or listening to music. Make sure that you don't fall asleep on the couch. When you find yourself becoming sleepy, return to your bedroom and attempt to sleep once again. Remember that this strategy should be repeated throughout the night. That is, every time you've been in bed awake for fifteen to twenty minutes, you need to get up and move to another location until you think you're sleepy enough to get to sleep.

E = ELIMINATE NAPS

Naps can be relaxing and possibly even enjoyable, and many people do feel the need for a rest in the afternoon. But these naps can be quite disruptive to nighttime sleeping, so it's best that you do not nap at all. If you are unable to avoid a nap in the middle of the day, be sure to limit your nap to one hour and do not sleep after 3:00 P.M.

P = PUT YOUR PLAN INTO ACTION

If you truly want to experience the benefits of stimulus-control training, it must become part of your lifestyle. You must consistently work toward learning new relationships between your bedroom and your behaviors. Over time, the principles highlighted here will become much more automatic.

Sleep Hygiene Training

Sleep hygiene refers to the process of improving sleep by focusing on your health practices and environmental influences. The goal of this intervention is to increase your awareness of how your health-related behaviors and certain environmental factors may be making it less likely that you will be able to get a quality night's rest and to teach you how to change these circumstances to benefit your sleep. Sleep hygiene involves following six simple rules (Morin 1993).

First, the use of caffeine should be discontinued at least four to six hours before going to bed. Caffeine is a stimulant that is found in coffee, tea, soft drinks, chocolate, and even some over-the-counter allergy and cold medications. Caffeine alters your sleep and has been shown to increase the amount of time it takes you to fall asleep as well as the number of times you wake up during the night (Karacan et al. 1976).

Second, as nicotine is also a stimulant, it too should be avoided near bedtime. Although it is true that in mild doses nicotine may have relaxing and sedating effects, in moderate to high doses, nicotine serves to increase bodily arousal through increases in heart rate and respiratory rate. In an interesting study, it was noted that people who smoke more than a pack of cigarettes per day were more likely to have difficulties falling asleep compared with people who either were nonsmokers or smoked less than a pack a day (Kales et al. 1984). Thankfully, it also seems to be true that if you are able to successfully stop smoking, sleep quality can improve in a relatively short period of time (Soldatos et al. 1980). At the very least, if using nicotine (cigarettes, smokeless tobacco, pipe tobacco), it is extremely important to use it as far away from your bedtime as possible.

Third, the use of alcohol can cause substantial sleep problems. Alcohol is a depressant, and when consumed near bedtime it may very well have the effect of reducing the amount of time it takes you to fall asleep as well as help you to sleep very deeply during the initial stage of the night. However, as the night progresses, withdrawal will occur in the form of physiological arousal, experiences of anxiety, and perhaps gastrointestinal discomfort and nausea. Ultimately, alcohol really has the effect of disturbing and shortening your sleep, with substantial reductions in the deep sleep or delta wave sleep (stage 4) we mentioned earlier. Thus, like caffeine and nicotine use, if alcohol cannot be avoided entirely, it certainly should not be used within the four-hour window prior to bedtime.

Fourth, eating too much food before bedtime can cause sleep disruption. In particular, eating too much food has the effect of causing your digestive system to be extremely active. This activity can create disruptions in the amount of time it takes to fall asleep. On the other hand, there is reason to believe that a light snack before bedtime may actually help to improve sleep, although the precise reasons for this remain somewhat unclear. Like too much food intake, drinking too many fluids before bedtime can be related to decreased sleep quality in the form of more frequent nighttime awakenings and urges to urinate.

Fifth, it's also important to be sure not to exercise within the four-hour window prior to bedtime, as exercise increases bodily activity and speeds up your autonomic nervous system, causing increases in heart rate, respiratory rate, and so forth. We are all aware that exercise and physical fitness are important to health and well-being. Interestingly, as far as the effects of exercise on sleep, there is some good information to suggest that for people who are physically fit, exercise may help to decrease the time it takes to fall asleep and increase the duration of sleep (Morin 1993). Among unfit people, however, increased exercise can actually serve to disrupt sleep. However, as the benefits of a moderate exercise program are well known, we recommend moderate exercise (for example, three times per week for at least twenty minutes) for all people engaged in this workbook (of course, with recognition that cancer treatment and associated side effects may periodically limit your ability to exercise). So if you can engage in a moderate exercise program in the late afternoon, even if you presently are unfit and this exercise temporarily disrupts your sleep, in the long term you will be more healthy and also have a more restful night's sleep.

Finally, to improve the quality of your sleep, there are some commonsense environmental factors that need to be taken into account. Although some people may benefit from repetitive and soothing sounds (like soft music, a fan, or sound machines), for the most part, noise should be kept to a minimum. If too much noise is experienced that may be partially uncontrollable (a snoring bed partner, traffic), earplugs may be a useful solution. Too much light in your bedroom also might be problematic, but this can be resolved through heavier blinds or perhaps the use of an eye mask. Although people have slightly different preferences, room temperature and mattress firmness should also be considered. People generally sleep a little better when room temperatures are a little bit cooler, and, depending on individual circumstances that might include pain or other medical problems, desired mattress firmness may vary considerably.

SLEEP HYGIENE SUMMARY

1. Discontinue caffeine use at least four to six hours before bedtime.

2. Discontinue nicotine use at least four hours before bedtime.

3. Discontinue alcohol use at least four hours prior to bedtime.

4. Eat nothing or only a very small snack in the last few hours before bedtime.

5. Engage in a moderate exercise program, but be sure not to exercise within four hours of bedtime.

6. Consider how noise, light, room temperature, and your mattress may be affecting your sleep.

EXERCISE: MY SLEEP HYGIENE

After reading the preceding section on sleep hygiene, write about what your sleep hygiene is like. How well do you follow these rules? What kind of changes could you make to improve your sleep hygiene?

_____

_____

_____

_____

_____

_____

_____

Now that you have learned about stimulus control therapy and sleep hygiene, we ask that you practice these strategies consistently over the next two weeks. To remind yourself, you should probably add something like "practicing sleep" to your Master Activity Log and Behavior Checkout that you are using as part of behavioral activation. After two weeks have elapsed, complete your second and final sleep diary.

Date _____ to _____	Example	Mon	Tue	Wed	Thu	Fri	Sat	Sun
Yesterday, I napped from ____ to ____ (note the time of all naps).	12:00 to 1:30 P.M.							
Yesterday, I took ____ mg of medication and/or ____ oz of alcohol as a sleep aid.	Xanax .5 mg							
Last night, I went to bed and turned the lights off at ____ o'clock.	10:30							
After turning the lights out, I fell asleep in ____ minutes.	45 min							
My sleep was interrupted ____ times (specify number of nighttime awakenings).	2							
My sleep was interrupted for ____ minutes (specify duration of each awakening).	25, 35							
This morning, I woke up at ____ o'clock (note time of last awakening).	5:30							
This morning, I got out of bed at ____ o'clock (specify the time).	6:15							
When I got up this morning I felt ____ . (1=Exhausted, 5=Refreshed)	2							
Overall, my sleep last night was ____ . (1=Very Restless, 5=Very Sound).	2							

After completing your sleep training and this second sleep diary, what do you notice? How does this sleep diary look different from the sleep diary you completed prior to learning about stimulus-control therapy and sleep-hygiene training? Are you falling asleep more quickly? Are you waking up fewer times during the night? Are you taking fewer naps? Are you exercising more? Are you going to bed and waking up at the same time each day? Are your sleep ratings higher?

The exercises in the chapter should be very useful toward addressing any sleep problems you might have been experiencing. Getting a quality night's sleep is essential for restoring your body's energy supply and will help give you the strength you require to engage in your activation exercises. Feeling rested will also help you to be more engaged and effective in social situations and will assist you in having more rewarding social interactions. In an effort to further improve the quality of your social experiences, the next chapter will help you become a more effective communicator.

CHAPTER 9

Assertiveness and Social-Skills Training

TIME: Approximately One Week

One of the problems you may be experiencing that may stand in the way of obtaining greater pleasure in your life may be the way you relate to other people. It's one thing to suggest that you increase the frequency of your social contacts and another for you to actually experience satisfaction or pleasure in these social situations. Indeed, if you don't have the necessary social skills or you experience unusually high levels of social anxiety, these problems may greatly reduce the likelihood of obtaining pleasure in social situations and in fact might actually make you feel more anxious or depressed. Therefore, based on the work of other clinical researchers (Hope et al. 2000; Turner, Beidel, and Cooley-Quille 1997), the purpose of this chapter is to help you be a more effective communicator, be more assertive, and overcome social anxiety that may be negatively affecting your ability to socialize. Just as the other supplemental behavioral activation strategies may be useful to include in your behavioral plan, the skills you learn in this chapter can help you with all social activities you have included in your master activity log.

BECOMING A MORE EFFECTIVE COMMUNICATOR

On your path toward becoming a more effective social person, it will help to review some important information that relates to how you speak with people and how the things you say and the way you say them may determine whether a conversation is likely to continue and whether a relationship might develop. This next section presents useful ideas for beginning and maintaining conversations and also focuses on skills that will be important toward building high-quality friendships.

Initiating and Maintaining Conversation

The first step toward becoming a more effective communicator is learning how to initiate and maintain a conversation. When deciding to initiate a conversation, there are several important rules of thumb to keep in mind. For example, it probably would be a good idea to start a conversation under the following circumstances (Turner et al. 1997):

You get introduced to someone.

You keep seeing the same person.

You come across people you know in different situations (for instance, seeing your neighbor at your gym).

In contrast, it might not be the best idea to start a conversation with someone who appears to be busy or preoccupied, does not seem interested, as determined by noticing their nonverbal behaviors (no eye contact, head down, negative facial expression), or when the person is engaged in conversation with somebody else. Under other circumstances, it would be more appropriate for you to engage in conversation. For example, when the person offers a smile or kind facial expression, eye contact, and isn't engaged in another activity or conversation, this might suggest the person would be willing to engage you in conversation.

Assuming that another person looks to be willing to have a conversation with you, the next issue relates to what you say to the person. The answer to this question will partially depend upon the status of your relationship with that person. For example, if you already have a prior history with this person, it may be appropriate to begin your conversation by saying something like "Hi Mary, how are things going?" or "Hello John, I haven't seen you in a long time. What's new?" On the other hand, if you're initiating an interaction with a stranger, the stakes are a little bit higher in the sense that the outcome is a little less predictable. When you have a prior relationship with someone, you presumably know something about them, including being better able to judge whether or not they might be receptive to engaging you in conversation. With strangers, you generally know nothing about how interested they might be in beginning a conversation with you, whether or not they are a social person, or whether the person might be shy or perhaps just introverted and uncomfortable with meeting strangers. So this is definitely a higher-risk situation than approaching a prior acquaintance.

That does not mean, however, that pleasurable, interesting, and even relationship-building conversations cannot take place with strangers. On the contrary, most of the people in your life whom you consider to be good friends were at one time strangers. Therefore, at times it may be useful to attempt to engage strangers in conversation. Remember the discussion from chapter 5, when you learned that people generally behave to obtain or avoid something? What can be obtained or gained by engaging a stranger in conversation? Perhaps you will have an intellectually or emotionally stimulating conversation; perhaps you will learn more about the kinds of people you find more or less interesting; perhaps you will gain a sense of self-confidence from taking the risk of approaching someone you don't know; or maybe you will even develop a long-term friendship. It is important to keep in mind, however, that not all strangers you approach will want to develop a conversation with you. In these cases, remember not to take things too personally. You have no idea why someone is disinterested, and it doesn't mean that you are unworthy of conversation or an unlikable person. On the contrary, as stated before, among other things, the person may be shy, busy doing other things, too stressed to converse, or preoccupied in thoughts about other things.

So, if you do decide to approach a stranger to begin a conversation, what should you say? The most important thing to keep in mind is that you should be sure to smile and introduce yourself. Next, it's probably in your best interest to talk about something you have in common and to focus on a more general topic. For example, you might say, "I notice that both of us seem to be here each day at about the same time" or "Looks like we both enjoy the same coffee place" or "So how long has your son been playing soccer?" General topics of conversation might include sports, employment, community events, or even the weather. Also, remember that if you are interested in maintaining a conversation, it is always a good strategy to ask open-ended as opposed to closed-ended questions. *Open-ended questions* are questions that require the other person to respond with more than just a one word answer (yes or no). It is these types of questions that better allow for conversations to develop.

OPEN-ENDED QUESTIONS

What do you think about this soccer program?

What kind of hobbies do you like?

How do you feel about the new highway being constructed?

CLOSED-ENDED QUESTIONS

Do you like this soccer program?

Do you like to golf?

I don't like the idea of this highway being developed, do you agree?

Once you have initiated a conversation, it's important to be able to determine whether or not to continue the conversation. In other words, you need to be able to determine whether the person you are engaging is open to conversation. The more the person displays the following behaviors, the more likely it is that he or she is interested in having a conversation:

They smile at you.

They make frequent eye contact.

They don't appear preoccupied with other tasks or other people.

They respond to your questions and comments.

They provide responses that are more than yes or no answers.

They ask you questions.

Being aware of these behaviors can greatly increase the likelihood that you will have pleasurable social encounters. Finally, in an effort toward maintaining conversations, particularly with strangers, it's worth emphasizing two other points. First, try to avoid potentially sensitive and controversial topics such as politics, sex, alcohol and drugs, and so forth. Moving too quickly into these areas with people you are just meeting may come across as offensive and quickly destroy any chance you might have of establishing a meaningful relationship. Second, in trying to maintain conversations, it is important to be a good listener. This means being able to reflect back what another person is saying to you. For example, when meeting a stranger, you often learn some important information early in the conversation, such as the person's name and maybe something about their family or hobbies that they enjoy. Unfortunately, it is at the beginning of conversations where you are also most likely to be anxious and may not attend to this kind of information. So at the beginning of conversations, it is important to be aware of your anxiety and work very hard to pay close attention to what a person is telling you so that you may later reflect back to them that you know their name or are familiar with their interests or hobbies. Being able to communicate these things provides others with the impression that you are a good listener and are interested in what they have to say. These are qualities that people look for when they are deciding on whether or not to pursue friendships.

Learning to Establish and Maintain Friendships

Now that you are familiar with the basic skills involved with initiating and maintaining a conversation, it's time to move forward with learning how to establish and maintain enduring relationships. Before discussing some methods of how to do this, it's important that you have a good understanding of the type of person that you would like to have as a friend. People's needs are very different when it comes to deciding whether another person is more or less suitable as a friend. What are your needs?

EXERCISE: A DESCRIPTION OF MY IDEAL FRIEND

What would your ideal friend be like? What kind of qualities would he or she have to have? What would their behaviors have to be like? How would they act around you? What are you *not* looking for in a friend?

_____

_____

_____

_____

_____

_____

_____

Now that you have an idea of the type of friendship you're looking for, it's a good time to discuss how to go about finding this person and how to develop a meaningful relationship. The first major issue relates to where you go to find this friend. In general, you should strongly consider the places you go, as these are likely rewarding situations and experiences that you probably value and would also value in a friend. Among these places, any work-related function would seem to be a good place to meet people. Indeed, given that you already have your place of employment as a common topic by which to build conversation, you are already ahead of the game. Other potential places might include social functions and discussion groups held within the church, evening classes offered by high schools or colleges (something like carpentry, gardening, or cooking perhaps), health clubs or gymnasiums, or various community organizations (Turner et al. 1997). It's also possible that you will find an opportunity to develop a relationship during the course of your everyday activities, which may not include the more predictable situations just mentioned. For example, you could meet someone at the grocery store, at the shopping mall, at the bookstore or library, at the park, or any number of other places. Quite commonly, it is likely that you will have opportunities to meet other people through acquaintances that you already have developed.

After you have met someone, used your greeting and conversational skills presented earlier, and established that the person might be someone you are interested in spending more time with, it's time to invite that person to spend some time with you. There are really only three rules for inviting someone to join you in an activity. The first is that you generally ask a person to join you in a smaller activity that doesn't require a huge amount of time or monetary commitment. So a cup of coffee, a beer after work, or even a quick lunch would be suitable activities, whereas dinner and a movie, a trip to the amusement park, or a lengthy hike and a picnic would probably not be suitable. Second, it's always a good idea to present your request to spend more time in an "open" manner, such that the other person feels free to make a decision in a way that will not be offensive to you. Beginning your request with a word such as "maybe" or "perhaps" is always a good idea. So you might say "Maybe we could go for a cup of coffee sometime?" This type of request is better than saying "Let's go for a cup of coffee today" because if the person is disinterested, they are put into an awkward position of having to say no to someone they have just met. With the more preferred request, even if the person is disinterested, he or she can say something more along the lines of "We'll see" or "Thanks for the offer—let me think about it, if you would." Third, do not try to pressure people into engaging in activities if judging by their verbal (for example, saying no or "I'd rather not") or nonverbal behaviors (no eye contact, unfriendly posture), it appears as though they are disinterested.

If your request is effective and the person is interested in spending time with you, terrific. Make sure to ask the person about which days and times are better to meet, and try to schedule the activity. If the person does not express interest in spending time with you, try not to be offended and remember that there are plenty of other of people in the world who would jump at the chance. Politely thank the person for considering your request, and maybe even suggest that he let you know if he changes his mind about your offer.

If you manage to schedule an activity, follow through with it, and have a good time, remembering that this is only the beginning. Relationships take work, and you will need to think about ways that you can work to maintain your new friendship. There are many ways to maintain your friendship through regular contact, including communication through phone calls, text messaging, e-mail, face-to-face contact, and letters. In working toward maintaining your friendship, remember these few simple suggestions that will help you to continue to build on the relationship over time:

Maintain contact over regular intervals, the duration of which is acceptable to both parties.

Work together to decide which method of contact is most preferable.

When arguments or conflicts arise, do not avoid them, but rather work together to address and solve the problems.

Remember that compromise and respect are important components of a relationship.

When your relationship partner is doing something that really pleases you, be sure to let him or her know what that is.

Try to be dependable and reliable for your relationship partner.

Be loyal and honest with your friend.

Remember to be a good listener.

Be generous and make sacrifices on occasion.

Try to forgive whenever you can.

If your friend has fears or anxieties, try to relieve them.

If your friend needs help, try your best to be there.

Understand and accept that nobody is perfect and everyone makes mistakes.

EXERCISE: HOW I CAN BE A BETTER FRIEND

As you read through the preceding list, think about your past relationships with both women and men. What are some of your strengths as a friend? What are some of your weaknesses, and what do you need to work on?

_____

_____

_____

_____

_____

_____

_____

Learning How to Be More Assertive

Now that you have learned how to more effectively initiate and sustain conversations as well as how to develop more rewarding interpersonal relationships, we turn our attention to a problem that some people have in relationships, namely an inability to be assertive. The ability to be *assertive* refers to the process of standing up for personal rights and expressing thoughts, feelings, and beliefs in direct, honest, and appropriate ways that do not violate another person's rights. A lack of assertiveness skills can result in other people overstepping their boundaries with you, feelings that you have been taken advantage of, a decrease in self-esteem, and perhaps increased anxiety and depression. Therefore, in an effort to further increase your positive social experiences, if you aren't already assertive, it's time that you learned.

Assertive behavior is to be distinguished from an aggressive communication style. With an *aggressive* approach to interacting with others, you stand up for personal rights and express your thoughts, feelings, and beliefs as well. Even though this expression is typically honest in that you are expressing yourself based on an emotional experience (anger), the way you express it is usually inappropriate and often too reactive and tends to violate the rights of other people. Clearly, this is an ineffective method to communicate that more often than not can lead to increased aggressive behaviors by all parties involved.

When you are not assertive and not necessarily aggressive, your communication style may be considered too passive. With a *passive* communication style, you fail to express your feelings, thoughts, and beliefs and thereby do not allow others to understand your feelings or position on matters. This passivity may result in others violating your rights or taking advantage of you. People often behave passively so that they will be liked and accepted by other people or to avoid potential confrontations and conflict with people in their lives. There are many characteristics of passive behavior. These include a weak, soft, and often apologetic voice, poor eye contact, weak or stooped posture, and general nervousness. In contrast, the assertive communication style involves being firm yet relaxed in your conversational tone, having good eye contact and an attentive attitude, and a relaxed body posture that exudes confidence.

When you think about how you interact with other people, do you behave in ways that are assertive? Complete the following exercise to determine how assertive you are.

EXERCISE: HOW ASSERTIVE ARE YOU?

Check yes or no for each of the following questions:

Do you ask for help if you need it?	YES ____	NO ____
Do you express anger and annoyance appropriately?	YES ____	NO ____
Do you ask questions when you're confused?	YES ____	NO ____
Do you volunteer your opinions when you think or feel differently from others?	YES ____	NO ____
Do you speak up in public fairly frequently?	YES ____	NO ____
Are you able to say no when you don't want to do something?	YES ____	NO ____
Do you speak with a generally confident manner, communicating caring and strength?	YES ____	NO ____
Do you look at people when you're talking to them?	YES ____	NO ____

If you answered no to a couple of these questions, it may be that you are behaving too unassertively in social situations. As we mentioned, it's possible that your unassertive behavior may be related to fears or anxiety about being disliked or rejected by others. It also is very possible that you have learned to be unassertive, perhaps by growing up in a home where one or both of your parents were unassertive. It also is possible that you were once more assertive than you are today, but that someone in your life punished your assertive behavior by not attending to you, or even worse, acting aggressively toward you when you behaved assertively.

However, we want to assure you that for the most part, individuals respond favorably to someone who is assertive, so long as being assertive involves being respectful of the rights of other people. For instance, it's important that when you are assertive, you focus statements on someone's behavior rather than interpersonal qualities that they might have. For example, an assertive statement that focused on behavior would be "I do not like it when you yell at me. It frightens me and makes me want to be alone. Instead, please try to talk to me in a calm voice." In contrast, an unassertive and more antagonistic statement that focused on interpersonal qualities might be "I hate your anger and meanness. You're an annoying person." The latter statements involve the use of labeling someone and are much less likely to have the desired effect of reducing yelling behavior.

In fact, they could potentially make the situation even more conflictual. When learning how to be more assertive, it's often useful to follow this simple formula (fill in the blanks):

I feel _____ when you _____

because _____ . I want/need _____ .

So for example, you might say

I feel <u>hurt</u> when you <u>yell</u> because <u>it makes me feel unloved</u>. I want <u>you to talk to me in a calmer and more respectful voice</u>.

Now think of someone who you think you need to be more assertive toward and complete this sentence.

I feel _____ when you _____

because _____ . I want/need _____ .

The next time you have the opportunity, try using this assertive statement and see if it has the desired effect on the person's behavior.

Another point worth mentioning is that even assertive behavior is not always effective. Remember that you are learning assertiveness skills for your benefit and not necessarily for the purpose of changing other people. Being assertive will help you to feel better and help you to gain self-confidence, regardless of whether other people's behaviors change. Remember, while it is within your power to change your behavior (for example, to become more assertive), you cannot always change the behavior of other people. Sometimes this is simply beyond your control, and no amount of assertive behavior will change other people, particularly those who are stuck to a particular viewpoint or method of interacting. Therefore, control what you have the power to control—what you say and do when you are interacting with other people.

There are really two general circumstances where it will be most important for you to be assertive. These situations involve having to refuse unreasonable requests that are being made of you and asking other people to change their behavior. In both situations it's important to maintain direct eye contact, keep your posture open and relaxed, maintain a calm but direct voice, and be sure your facial expression agrees with the message. In both circumstances, in addition to possibly using the formula presented above, it might be helpful to begin with an apology. For example, for an unreasonable request, you might say, "I'm sorry, but I feel that there is no possible way I can complete both reports by the end of the working day." Next, it is important to provide a brief explanation for why you are refusing the request, such as "The reason I will not be able to finish both is because I had the project proposal this afternoon, which took a substantial amount of time." Finishing up with a statement about what it would take to complete the request is always a good idea, something to the effect of "I would be pleased to do both reports, but having a little more notice next time would help me to make the deadline." When requesting that someone change their behavior, in addition to using the above formula, always remember to indicate to the other person how you would like them to behave the next time a similar situation arises.

EXERCISE: REFUSING AN UNREASONABLE REQUEST

Think about the last time somebody made an unreasonable request of you. What was it?

_____

_____

What did you do?

_____

_____

What could you say next time? Remember to use the apology strategy, provide a brief reason why you are refusing the request, and state what would be necessary for you to complete the request.

_____

_____

_____

_____

_____

_____

_____

_____

LEARNING TO MANAGE YOUR SOCIAL ANXIETY

While working on your social skills can improve the quality of your social interactions and thus create a more rewarding lifestyle, the pleasure of interacting with someone (or a group of people) can be dampened if you feel too anxious in social situations. As we presented in chapter 3, the extreme form of social anxiety, or feeling highly tense or nervous around others, is referred to as social phobia. Remember that with social phobia, social situations often are avoided entirely; or if you do approach social situations, you may experience extreme distress until the interaction is over. Strong physiological symptoms, negative thoughts, and fears of doing something humiliating or embarrassing are also common with this problem.

As you also learned earlier, people with cancer may develop symptoms of social phobia as a consequence of illness-related experiences (for instance, receiving a mastectomy for breast cancer, having fears associated with bladder or colorectal cancer, or having side effects of chemotherapy such as hair loss and dry skin). When people are excessively anxious around others, social interactions and gatherings that once were pleasurable can become almost intolerable and even depressing. Therefore, because you know how important social support can be toward living a more fulfilling life (recall chapter 1) and helping you to cope with your cancer experience, social anxiety is something that you must work toward overcoming.

So when you are developing your behavioral hierarchy (chapter 5), two recommendations are important to consider. First, you should definitely work toward developing your social system through including social behaviors and experiences. Second, if these social experiences are anxiety provoking, this problem needs to be addressed. If you seem to have some of the symptoms of social anxiety we outlined earlier in this book, this section will be useful to read and incorporate into your lifestyle and behavioral hierarchy. For example, in addition to including goals on your behavioral hierarchy such as spending more time with a certain friend, going to social gatherings with your spouse or partner, or calling a friend on the telephone, you may want to include a goal of working through social anxiety. This section will provide the basis by which to accomplish this goal.

GRADUATED EXPOSURE TO SOCIAL SITUATIONS

To overcome your fear of any situation, the most important thing to do is to learn how to face that situation and to learn that what you fear will not necessarily happen. For example, if a child is afraid of the dark and is scared that the boogeyman might come get him in bed, the way he will overcome this fear will be to continually face this situation and learn that no matter how dark it is, what time it is, or whether mother or father is in the room, the boogeyman will not come get him in bed. As another example, if you have cancer, have lost your hair as a result of chemotherapy, and are fearful others will not accept you because of hair loss, the way to overcome this fear is to spend time with other people and learn that you are accepted regardless of whether you have your hair.

Exposure refers to the process of coming into contact with your fears. In other words, you spend more time in situations that cause you to feel fearful or anxious so that you will learn to feel more comfortable in these situations. A big part of exposing yourself to your fears involves building up your self-confidence so that you feel capable of coping with the situations that cause you fear or anxiety. Just as any other skill, exposure is best learned gradually. Think about lifting weights. When you are beginning to lift weights, you would generally begin with lighter weights so that you could build up some initial strength. Over time, as you become stronger and stronger, you could increase the amount of weight that you are lifting. Well, one way to think about exposure is that you will be engaged in the process of building up your mental as opposed to physical strength. The way to do this is to identify social situations that cause you to feel anxious, then gradually work up to situations causing the highest anxiety levels.

Before providing you with specific guidelines for how to engage in social exposure, it's important that you understand why exposure works (Hope et al. 2000). First of all, when you are socially anxious it is very common to experience a number of physical symptoms that might include increased heart rate, difficulty breathing, sweating, and shaking. When socially anxious people are in a social situation, often these symptoms will occur and the person will sometimes address this problem by escaping the social situation. This strategy effectively stops the physical symptoms, but the person never learns that the symptoms would go away naturally if only they stayed in the social situation and got more practice.

Habituation refers to the process where physical symptoms decrease over time with continued contact with a feared situation or object. Habituation is much more likely to occur as you expose yourself regularly to what makes you anxious. So in the case of social situations, the more you come into contact with people and the more time you spend with people, the more the intensity and duration of your anxiety will diminish. The key is giving yourself the opportunity to learn that if you stay in a social situation long enough, eventually your heart will stop pounding, your legs will stop shaking, and your sweating will stop—all without having to escape from the situation.

A second reason that exposure is effective is that behaving differently allows you to have different experiences, which in turn allows you to change the way you think about the world. For example, when you put yourself in social situations, you may see and learn that other people are not going to evaluate you critically, make fun of you, or treat you like you are an insignificant or unworthy human being. Having this kind of experience will enable you to gain confidence in social situations, teach you that your beliefs about other people may not be accurate, decrease your anxiety, and, perhaps most importantly, increase the chances that you will be more likely to engage in social behaviors in the future.

Beginning the Process of Social Exposure: Constructing a Fear Hierarchy

The first step in learning to overcome your social anxiety through exposure is to develop your fear hierarchy. A *fear hierarchy* is a detailed list of those social situations that cause you to feel the symptoms of social anxiety (such as physical symptoms, negative thoughts, and a desire to escape or avoid). In constructing this fear hierarchy, it is important to think hard about any and all situations where you experience social anxiety. Here is an example of what a fear hierarchy might look like:

SOCIAL SITUATION	RANK
Talking within a group of people	2
Saying a prayer at the dinner table	11
Giving a speech in public	1

Talking to a member of the opposite sex	4
Writing a check in front of someone	12
Having dinner at someone's house	6
Talking to your boss	3
Talking with a friend on the phone	10
Talking to an unfamiliar person on the phone	7
Having to ask someone for directions	9
Attending a party	5
Meeting with a friend to do something together	8

EXERCISE: YOUR FEAR HIERARCHY

Now it is your turn to build your fear hierarchy. Think carefully about the situations that cause you to experience social anxiety, and write these situations down in the table below. If you are having difficulty thinking about specific situations, consider the following (Hope et al. 2000):

> Speaking in front of a group

>> Large vs. small group

>> Familiar vs. unfamiliar people

> Being the center of attention

> Casual conversations

>> Friend vs. acquaintance vs. stranger

> Meeting someone new

>> Man vs. woman

> Eating or drinking in front of others

> Writing or typing while being observed

> Being assertive

> Answering the telephone

> Talking with an authority figure

> Talking with an attractive person

> Job interviews

> Taking communion at church

> Unexpectedly seeing an acquaintance

> Giving or receiving a compliment

Attending meetings

    For work

    With teachers

    For a community organization

SOCIAL SITUATION	RANK

Now, looking back at the sample fear hierarchy, rank your situations. The situation that causes you the most anxiety, is most difficult to engage in, and might be avoided most frequently should be given a rank of 1 ("giving a speech in public" on the sample hierarchy). Count up to the situation on your list that causes you the least anxiety (for instance, "writing a check in front of someone" on the sample hierarchy).

Engaging in Exposure

Now that you have constructed your fear hierarchy, you are ready to begin your first exposure session. There are two strategies that you will use to engage in exposure—imaginal and in-vivo exposure. *Imaginal exposure* refers to the process of exposing yourself to your feared situations through your imagination, and *in-vivo exposure* refers to exposing yourself to your feared situations in real life. For each of the items on your fear hierarchy, you will begin by exposing yourself imaginally, then work your way toward approaching the situation in real life. Beginning to confront your fears through your imagination first allows you to approach your situations in a less anxiety-provoking way than if you were actually directly faced with the situation in real life.

So, let's take the least anxiety provoking situation on your fear hierarchy. Let's say that this situation involves talking to a friend on the phone. The first step in doing imaginal exposure is to make sure your environment is going to allow you to focus. Therefore, it is best if you conduct imaginal exposure in a quiet and relaxed setting. It's best if you have a comfortable chair and a dimly lit room, with as little noise as possible in the background. If you have children, it is probably wise to arrange your time so that you can conduct your exposure sessions when they are at school, asleep, or otherwise occupied. Make sure you are wearing comfortable clothing, and if you wear glasses, it may be helpful to take them off.

DEVELOPING YOUR EXPOSURE SCENE

Now that you know when and where you will conduct your imaginal exposure sessions, it's time to focus on developing your exposure scene. In the case of talking to your friend on the phone, you would want to think about where you would be (in your home), who would initiate the call, how the conversation would start, what the topic of conversation might be, and how the conversation might end. Also, it is important to think about any physical symptoms of anxiety that you might have as well as some worrisome thoughts that might be associated with the situation. Some people even find it helpful to write these details down so they are consistent from one exposure session to the next. Remember that it is best if you do not try to avoid your bodily sensations or negative thoughts. Rather, as with the rest of this workbook, the goal is to approach and confront the situations, physical sensations, and negative thoughts that are causing you problems, learning to cope with and overcome these situations and symptoms.

WORKING THROUGH THE SCENE

Once you have decided on an appropriate place and time to conduct your imaginal exposure and have developed your scene, it is time to engage in the exposure. When you do this, you will get situated, close your eyes, and imagine the situation of talking to your friend in as much detail as possible without avoiding certain images, feelings, or thoughts that might be associated with talking to your friend on the phone. In other words, allow yourself to fully experience your anxiety. When you have finished imagining the entire scene, rate your experience on the subjective units of discomfort scale (SUDS).

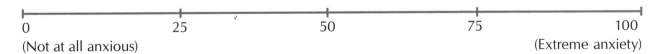

0   25   50   75   100

(Not at all anxious)   (Extreme anxiety)

You should record your rating and then close your eyes and repeat the imaginal exposure, using the exact same scene you just imagined. (Note: if you have difficulty imagining the scene and details of the scene, some people find it helpful to write down the specific details of the scene and then make an audio recording that they can play back over and over.) This process should continue until there is a 50 percent reduction in your initial SUDS score. So, if you recorded a SUDS score of 90 after your first exposure, you would continue with your imaginal exposure until you reached a score of 45. It is imperative that you continue with the imaginal exposure sessions until this reduction is reached. Initial sessions may take over an hour, but you can expect the duration of these sessions to decrease over time. It also is critical that you engage in the imaginal exposure exercise at least once a day. Remember that your goal is to habituate to a situation so that it no longer creates the same anxiety that you once experienced. Repetitive and consistent practice will allow this to happen at a quicker pace.

IN-VIVO EXPOSURE

Once you are finding that your imaginal scene is no longer creating the same level of initial anxiety (for example, you start at 50 instead of 90) or that you are habituating much quicker than normal (say, an imaginal exposure session that lasts ten minutes instead of an hour), you are ready to do the in-vivo (or real-life) exposure. Put simply, this involves actually picking up the phone and contacting your friend. Your imaginal practice will have prepared you well to follow through with this task, but you can still probably expect to experience some degree of anxiety, as this is a real-world experience that will be somewhat different from what has been occurring in your imagination. That's okay. The most important thing to do is to not be controlled by your anxiety. When conversing with your friend on the phone, it is perfectly understandable that you may feel somewhat anxious. Do not end the conversation prematurely or try to escape from the situation. Just as you learned from your imaginal exposure practice, remember that your anxiety will eventually pass if you just stick with the situation for a long enough period of time. As with imaginal exposure, you want to be able to practice in-vivo exposure on a regular basis so that you will have a chance to habituate to real-world experiences. However, you also probably don't want to call the same friend several times a day. Therefore, it will be important for you to be creative. In this situation, for example, identifying several friends or acquaintances that can serve this purpose would be useful.

CONTINUED PRACTICE

When you feel you have mastered the least anxiety provoking social scene on your hierarchy and are no longer experiencing a high level of anxiety, it is time for you to move on to the next social scene. Again, remember to start each new scene with imaginal exposure practice first, followed by in-vivo exposure. Also remember that a substantial portion of social anxiety may be related to problems with social skills and a lack of confidence in your ability to behave around other people. Recall that the social skills addressed earlier in this chapter may be useful in helping you to be more effective in social situations and also might help to significantly reduce your social anxiety. When you have successfully completed exposing yourself to all the situations on your fear hierarchy, your social anxiety should be greatly diminished, and your ability to experience more reward and pleasure in your life should be enhanced substantially.

CHAPTER 10

Relaxation, Mindfulness, and Self-Hypnosis

As you are working through chapter 5 and trying to determine which behaviors are going to be most useful for you to include on your Master Activity Log and Behavior Checkout, you may want to include relaxation practice, mindfulness, or self-hypnosis. Each of these strategies has been demonstrated to be useful toward improving a person's psychological well-being. For example, relaxation strategies have been shown to be useful for reducing anxiety symptoms and as a strategy for pain management (Barlow 2002). Mindfulness approaches have been helpful in reducing symptoms of pain, stress, anxiety, depression, and disordered eating behaviors (Baer 2003; Kristeller and Hallett 1999; Teasdale et al. 2000). Self-hypnosis has provided people with relief from anxiety and pain symptoms (Hawkins 2001). Although all these strategies may be helpful to you and certain similarities exist among them, different people often exhibit a preference for one approach over another. With this in mind, we encourage you to read this chapter and think about which strategy might be most appealing to you and then incorporate this approach into your behavioral plan (chapter 5) if you think this would be useful.

PROGRESSIVE MUSCLE RELAXATION

There are a number of different muscle-relaxation strategies and exercises that have been used to assist people with anxiety, depression, and pain problems (Barlow 2002; Craske, Barlow, and O'Leary 1992; Martin and Pear 1992). Indeed, people can be quite creative in finding ways to relax, including listening to music, watching a favorite television show or movie, going for a walk or jog, sitting in the park, and a countless number of other activities. While you may want to include one or a few of these behaviors in your Master Activity Log, you also might want to consider a relaxation strategy that is often used by mental health practitioners, called progressive muscle relaxation.

Progressive muscle relaxation refers to a tensing and relaxing strategy that is used to promote both physical and mental relaxation (Craske et al. 1992). The physical relaxation component involves practicing a series of tensing and relaxing exercises using many different muscles in your body. The mental relaxation component focuses more on the different sensations and experiences you have while you are tensing and relaxing certain muscle groups.

The progressive muscle relaxation strategy will initially take you approximately twenty-five to thirty minutes, though with repeated practice, you should eventually be able to go directly to the final step to achieve complete muscle relaxation. Remember that as with any new skill, progressive muscle relaxation will take time to learn. So try to be patient and know that eventually you will become skilled enough so that it will take you a short period of time (only one step) to achieve deep relaxation. This will be an important goal to achieve, because as you will see, learning progressive muscle relaxation initially involves twenty steps. Although this longer process is fine when it comes to learning how to relax in the comfort of your home, when you are in the "real world" and begin to experience anxiety, it will be more beneficial to you if relaxation can be achieved in a much shorter period of time.

Learning progressive muscle relaxation will be important to you for a few reasons. First, when you control your physical tension, you will be less likely to feel stressed and have a greater ability to control your worrying. Second, when you experience increased physical tension, these feelings can be highly uncomfortable and can be associated with whatever situation you are currently involved in (for instance, a social situation, work, school, or church). When this situation happens, you may experience a desire to escape from (and avoid) this situation to reduce feelings of anxiety or tension, and you have already learned that avoidance behavior only prolongs your problems. Learning how to relax more effectively can help to prevent these patterns from developing. Third, if you are experiencing symptoms of pain, increased muscle tension can serve to worsen these symptoms. Therefore, learning how to better relax your muscles also may help you to feel less pain.

If you decide to include relaxation as part of your behavioral plan, it will be important to make it a regular part of your daily routine, preferably at the same time and in a quiet environment where you will be free from distractions. If you are the type of person who suggests that you don't have time to relax, try to think about how this time pressure may be contributing to your feelings of anxiety and depression. In other words, make finding time for muscle relaxation a priority in your life. Odds are that you will find that learning this strategy may help to decrease those feelings of time pressure that you have been experiencing.

Progressive muscle relaxation really involves a structured procedure where you repeatedly tense and then relax different muscle groups in your body. The reason why you engage in this process is to learn the difference between when your muscles are tensed and when they are relaxed. As you will see, there is quite a dramatic difference in your body and muscle tone when you are relaxed versus when you are tense. The importance of learning this distinction is that you will be better equipped to recognize when you are beginning to feel tense. Being more aware of building tension in your body can serve as a cue to use your new relaxation skills and thereby break the anxiety cycle before it spirals out of control.

You may be a person who experiences substantial pain in one or more areas of your body. Even though you will be tensing many different muscles in your body, progressive muscle relaxation was not intended to produce any pain via this tensing procedure. Therefore, if there are certain parts of your body that are causing you pain, only tense these body parts to a degree that is comfortable. If pain in an area of your body is in fact excruciating, you may not even want to tense that body part at all during the procedure. Instead, just do the relaxing component when you get to this part of your body, and remember that learning how to relax body parts surrounding this area may have the added benefit of reducing tension and pain overall.

Engaging in Progressive Muscle Relaxation

Read through the following instructions carefully one time. Then go through them again, recording them as you go. If you think it might be too distracting to hear your own voice on a recording, ask your partner or a friend to help you with this task. When engaging in the relaxation exercise, simply play the recording back to yourself and follow the instructions. Remember to make sure you are in a comfortable chair, perhaps a recliner or a comfortable couch, and that there are few distractions that might interfere with the relaxation procedure. If you wear glasses, please remember to remove them before you begin.

RELAXATION INSTRUCTIONS

Record the following instructions, playing them back to achieve deep muscle relaxation (Martin and Pear 1992). General guidelines for implementing this program are as follows:

When developing the recording, use your voice in a way that is consistent with the instructions. Your voice should be slightly louder and rougher when reading the tensing instructions and softer and more soothing when reading the relaxation instructions.

Practice the entire twenty steps every day for at least one week.

After the first week, make a new recording of steps 1, 8, 15, and 20. Use this new recording for at least one week.

Make a new recording of only steps 1 and 20. Use this one for at least one week.

Step 1. Listen closely to these instructions. They will help to increase your ability to relax. Each time I pause, continue doing what you were doing before the pause. Now close your eyes and take three deep breaths. *Pause for ten seconds.*

Step 2. Make a tight fist with your left hand. Squeeze it tightly. Note how it feels. *Pause for five seconds.* Now relax. *Pause for five seconds.*

Step 3. Once again, squeeze your hand tightly and study the tension that you feel. *Pause for five seconds.* And once again, just relax and think of the tension disappearing from your fingers. *Pause for ten seconds.*

Step 4. Make a tight fist with your right hand. Squeeze it as tightly as you can, and note the tension in your fingers, your hand, and your forearm. *Pause for five seconds.* Now relax. *Pause for five seconds.*

Step 5. Once again, squeeze your right fist tightly and focus on the tension. *Pause for five seconds.* And again, just relax, allowing the tension to exit out of your hand and through your fingertips. *Pause for ten seconds.*

Step 6. Make a tight fist with your left hand and bend your arm to make your biceps hard. Hold it tense. *Pause for five seconds.* Now relax totally. Feel the warmth escape down your biceps, through your forearm, and out of your fingers. *Pause for ten seconds.*

Step 7. Now make a tight fist with the other hand and raise your hand to make your right biceps hard. Hold it tightly and feel the tension. *Pause for five seconds.* Now relax. Concentrate on the feelings flowing through your arm. *Pause for ten seconds.*

Step 8. Now, squeeze both fists at once and bend both arms to make them totally tense throughout. Hold it, and think about the tension you feel. *Pause for five seconds.* Now relax, and feel the total warmth and relaxation flowing through your muscles. All the tension is flowing out of your fingertips. *Pause for ten seconds.*

Step 9. Now, wrinkle your forehead and squint your eyes very tight and hard. Squeeze them tight and hard. Feel the tension across your forehead and through your eyes. Now relax. Note the sensations running through your eyes. Just relax. *Pause for ten seconds.*

Step 10. Okay, now squeeze your jaws tightly together and raise your chin to make your neck muscles hard. Hold it, bite down hard, tense your neck, and squeeze your lips really tight. *Pause for five seconds.* Now relax. *Pause for ten seconds.*

Step 11. Now, all together, wrinkle up your forehead and squeeze your eyes tight, bite down hard with your jaws, raise your chin and tighten up your neck, and make your lips tight. Hold them all and feel the tension throughout your forehead and eyes and jaw and neck and lips. Hold it. Now relax. Just totally relax and enjoy the tingling sensations. *Pause for ten seconds.*

Step 12. Now, squeeze both your shoulders forward as hard as you can until you feel your muscles pulling tightly right across your back, especially in the area between your shoulder blades. Squeeze them. Hold them tight. Now relax. *Pause for ten seconds.*

Step 13. Now squeeze your shoulders forward again and, at the same time, suck your stomach in as far as you can and tense your stomach muscles. Feel the tension throughout your stomach. Hold it. *Pause for five seconds.* Now relax. *Pause for ten seconds.*

Step 14. Once more, squeeze your shoulder blades forward again, suck in your stomach as far as you can, tense your stomach muscles, and feel the tension throughout your upper body. Now relax. *Pause for ten seconds.*

Step 15. Now, we are going to review all of the muscle systems that we have covered so far. First, take three deep breaths. *Pause for ten seconds.* Ready? Tighten up both fists and bend both of your arms to squeeze your biceps tight. Wrinkle your forehead and squeeze your eyes tight. Bite down hard with your jaws, raise your chin, and hold your lips tight. Squeeze your shoulders forward and suck in your stomach. Hold them all. Feel the tremendous tension throughout. Now relax. Take a deep breath. Just feel the tension disappearing. Think about the total relaxation throughout all of your muscles. In your arms, in your head, in your shoulders, and in your stomach. Just relax. *Pause for ten seconds.*

Step 16. Now, let's go to your legs. Focus on your left leg, particularly in your thigh and your calf. Tense your left thigh and left calf as tight as you can. Feel the pressure building, and notice the tension. *Pause for five seconds.* Now relax. *Pause for ten seconds.*

Step 17. Now, one more time, focus on your left thigh and calf, and tense these muscles as tight as you can. *Pause for five seconds.* Now relax. *Pause for ten seconds.*

Step 18. Now turn your focus on your right leg, particularly your thigh and your calf. Tense your right thigh and right calf as tight as you can. Feel the pressure building and notice the tension. *Pause for five seconds.* Now relax. *Pause for ten seconds.*

Step 19. Now let's do both legs together. Concentrating on both legs, squeeze the muscles in your thighs and calves as hard as you can. Feel the tension and pressure. *Pause for five seconds.* Now, let it all go and completely relax the muscles in your legs, enjoying the pleasant sensations of feeling relaxed. *Pause for fifteen seconds.*

Step 20. Now, take three deep breaths. *Pause for ten seconds.* Now tense all the muscles as they are named, exactly as you have practiced: Left fist and biceps, right fist and biceps, forehead, eyes, jaw, neck, lips, shoulders, stomach, left leg, right leg. Hold it. *Pause for five seconds.* Now relax. *Pause for ten seconds.* Breathe in deeply three times and then repeat the total tensing and then the total relaxing, and while you are breathing in deeply and then tensing and then relaxing, notice how relaxed all of your muscles feel. Now tense. *Pause for five seconds.* And relax. *Pause for five seconds.* Now, breathe normally and enjoy the completely tension-free state of your body and muscles. *Pause for thirty seconds.*

MINDFULNESS TRAINING

A second strategy that can be useful in managing your anxiety and depression, in terms of these emotions and the thoughts, physical symptoms, and behaviors that are associated with them, is mindfulness training. *Mindfulness* is a concept that has its roots in Eastern religions such as Buddhism and refers to a state of being attentive to and aware of what is taking place in the present. Moreover, this attention and awareness takes place on a level where a person just experiences and observes and is essentially nonjudgmental or nonevaluative about what they are experiencing. At this stage of research, it is clear that individuals differ quite substantially in their ability to be aware of and maintain attention to the present, and to be nonevaluative (Brown and Ryan 2003; Hayes, Strosahl, and Wilson 1999; Kabat-Zinn 2003). Important to this discussion, it is necessary to distinguish between the concepts of awareness and attention. Both terms are associated with the broader term of consciousness. *Awareness* refers to the background of what is going on in your life and what you are capable of sensing at any given moment in time. It is quite possible for someone to be very aware of something going on in their environment without being overly attentive to it. *Attention* is the process by which you focus your awareness onto something specific that is happening around you at a particular time. For example, if you are at a social gathering, you may be aware of where your friend is in the room, where the bar and stereo system are located, the sounds of people talking and music playing, and the scents of the hors d'oeuvres permeating the air. However, you may be attentive to, or intensely focused on, a conversation you are having with your business partner. Mindfulness is considered an enhanced attention to and awareness of current experience or present reality (Brown and Ryan 2003).

Why Mindfulness Is Important

Being mindful is associated with living in the moment and being aware of your surroundings, and therefore this practice has several important benefits. For example, people who are more mindful may be:

Better able to express their needs and concerns

Better able to identify conflict as it is developing

More equipped to obtain factual information from others

More in tune with their behaviors and the effect of their behaviors on other people

More in touch with their (and others') emotional experiences

Less likely to engage in automatic thoughts, habits, and unhealthy behavior patterns

Less likely to develop problems with depression and anxiety

In contrast to the advantages of being more mindful, not being aware and attentive to what is going on in your life, sometimes referred to as *mindlessness*, may have negative consequences. For example, not being attentive and present focused can provide a basis for engaging in rumination or excessive worrying or absorption in past experiences as well as make you more inclined to get caught up with anxiety or worry about the future. Additionally, not being mindful can create situations where your attention is so divided that you are engaged in multiple tasks or thinking about multiple aspects of your life simultaneously, making it virtually impossible to stay focused and be effective in whatever task is taking place in the present. Finally, mindlessness is strongly associated with a process called experiential avoidance. *Experiential avoidance* is defined as a person's unwillingness to remain in contact with or experience particular private events that might include bodily sensations, emotions, thoughts, and memories, as well as a tendency to avoid certain situations or events. Consistent with our earlier statements (chapters 4 and 5) that behavioral avoidance doesn't do much to improve your psychological health, a good body of research now exists that shows experiential avoidance is harmful to psychological well-being (Hayes et al. 1996). Therefore, being more mindful allows you to more fully experience your life and may protect you from developing psychological problems.

Research on Mindfulness Interventions

Research evaluating the effectiveness of various mindfulness-based psychological interventions has been nicely summarized (Baer 2003). Although the concept of mindfulness is an element of a number of different forms of therapy, it is perhaps most evident in two forms of therapy, mindfulness-based stress reduction (MBSR; Kabat-Zinn 1982) and mindfulness-based cognitive therapy (MBCT; Segal, Williams, and Teasdale 2002). Within these approaches, a number of different mindfulness meditation skills are taught, one of which we will present shortly for you to practice.

In the context of treating pain problems, MBSR was effectively used to reduce pain by having pain patients learn to carefully focus attention on pain sensations and to develop a nonjudgmental attitude toward these sensations and thoughts associated with pain. In other words, the objective was to have patients experience and accept pain symptoms without conscious and concentrated efforts to try to force the pain away. In addition to pain-related problems, MBSR and MBCT have shown very promising results as treatments for anxiety and panic problems (Kabat-Zinn et al. 1992), binge eating problems (Kristeller and Hallett 1999), and depression (Kabat-Zinn et al. 1992; Teasdale et al. 2000). In addition, mindfulness-based strategies also have been shown to have benefits for individuals with certain medical problems, including fibromyalgia and psoriasis (Baer 2003). Most importantly for you, MBSR has also been demonstrated as useful in reducing mood disturbance and stress levels among cancer patients (Brown and Ryan 2003; Speca et al. 2000).

How You Can Incorporate Mindfulness into Your Life

As with progressive muscle relaxation, mindfulness is a skill that requires practice. The decision of whether to include one or both of these strategies in your behavioral plan is entirely your choice. As you will recognize, although both procedures are designed to bring about reductions in feelings of anxiety, depression, and pain, the methods used are somewhat different. For example, with progressive muscle relaxation there is an active component of tensing and relaxing your muscles, and learning to discriminate between these two states can be very useful to you in the sense of learning to be more aware of your body's reactions and stress level. With mindfulness training, there is no focus on tensing muscles in the body, but there is more of an emphasis on cultivating a sense of peacefulness that is characterized by a focus on the present and an intense awareness of and attention to what is presently going on within you and around you. So, with progressive muscle relaxation, you learn to recognize and distinguish between two bodily states, and with mindfulness training, you learn to recognize your thoughts, feelings, and emotions in a broader manner. Both strategies can result in the same outcome, namely reductions in anxiety, depression, and pain—but through different mechanisms. Importantly, if you are the type of person who experiences a significant degree of pain, whether or not it is related to your cancer, mindfulness training might be the preferred option for you as it doesn't require you to work your muscles intensely.

ENGAGING IN MINDFULNESS TRAINING

Read the following instructions carefully, and then make a recording of these instructions. Once you have recorded the exercise, it will take approximately twenty minutes to complete, and most preferably you will be able to find time to complete the exercise on a daily basis. Just as with the progressive muscle relaxation exercise, if you think it will be too distracting to hear your own voice on a recording, ask your partner or a friend to help you with this task. When engaging in the mindfulness-training exercise, simply play the recording back to yourself and follow the instructions. Remember to make sure you find a comfortable seat in a place where you will not be distracted. Sit on the floor, perhaps putting a cushion underneath you, with your back upright and unsupported, if possible.

Mindfulness instructions. This is the body-awareness exercise. For this exercise, find a position either seated comfortably with your neck supported or lying down. You may wish to loosen any belts, take off your glasses, and just check in to make sure that your body is comfortable. As we go through this exercise, keep in mind an attitude of accepting whatever happens—in other words, of not trying to make anything happen, but just being present with what is, without judging your experience. You may find throughout this exercise that your mind wanders, that your mind is filled with thoughts, and whenever that happens, gently notice that your mind has wandered and then bring your mind back to the exercise.

To begin with, find your breath going in and out of your body, and spend a moment just feeling the sensation of breath, going in, going out … feeling your abdomen rising and falling, feeling the contact points of your body against the floor or in the chair and beginning to draw your attention to sensations within your body. *Pause for ten seconds.* The purpose of the exercise is to notice the feelings of your body without trying to change them and without judging. So now we will begin going through the body with gentle awareness. *Pause for five seconds.* First, draw your attention down to your right foot. *Pause for five seconds.* If you wish, you can use your breath, breathing in, imagining that your breath goes down into your right foot, bringing with it a gentle sensation of awareness, noticing whatever it is you feel in your toes, in the sole of your foot, in your heel. You may feel nothing at all, and that's okay. You may feel tension, warmth, coldness. Whatever it is, simply notice it with each breath, feeling your foot. *Pause for ten seconds.*

And now, letting your attention move through your ankle and into your right lower leg, notice sensations in your calf muscles and your shin. *Pause for five seconds.* Just watch whatever is going on there, using your breath to draw your attention. Try not to actually visualize your leg, but to feel it from the inside. *Pause for five seconds.* Let attention move now to your right knee (*pause for five seconds*), and then feel your right thigh, just noticing sensation in your thigh muscles. *Pause for five seconds.* If your mind is wandering, let the thoughts float away and bring your attention gently back with kindness to the feelings in your right thigh. And now, shifting attention to your left side … allow your breath to draw attention down to your left foot and notice all the sensations in your left foot, in your toes, in the sole of your foot, your heel, and arch, the top of your foot, allowing your awareness to take in whatever is there without judging it. *Pause for ten seconds.* And then, allow awareness to move to your left ankle. *Pause for five seconds.* Feel any sensations of tension or relaxation, letting awareness move to your left leg (*pause for five seconds*), feeling the muscles in your left calf (*pause for five seconds*), feeling the sensations in your left knee. *Pause for five seconds.* Gently draw your attention to your left thigh now. *Pause for five seconds.* Notice any sensation (*pause for five seconds*) … just letting it be what it is, bringing your attention gently back to this moment and to the sensations you are feeling. Feeling both of your legs, and now gently moving awareness into your pelvis, feeling your buttocks, your genitals, your hips, breathing awareness into the cradle of your pelvis, noticing any sensations of energy, any tension, just noticing, just holding all sensation in your awareness. *Pause for ten seconds.* Then, move to your lower back, feeling any tension in the lower muscles surrounding your spine … any pain, any achiness, using your breath to surround this sensation with accepting awareness. *Pause for ten seconds.* And then moving your attention to your belly, your abdomen, allowing your breath to move deeply into your abdomen … becoming aware of the multitude of activity within your vital organs, just breathing openness and space into the center of your abdomen, noticing whatever you notice. *Pause for fifteen seconds.* Now, move your attention up to your chest area, feeling your heart and your lungs … breathing into your chest space with great tenderness, just feeling whatever sensation is being held in that space, allowing for whatever sensation, whatever emotion you notice as you bring awareness to your heart center. *Pause for ten seconds.* Now, bring attention to your upper back and to the muscles of your shoulder blades and your shoulders, a place where we all carry tension, and notice what you feel in your shoulders … without trying to change it, just welcoming sensation within your awareness, breathing gently into your shoulders and your upper back. *Pause for ten seconds.* And now, allow awareness to move gradually down your right arm, feeling your upper arm, your triceps muscle, and moving slowly through your elbow, your lower right arm, feeling your wrist and the back of your hand, feeling the palm of your right hand, your fingers, allowing awareness to extend right down to your fingertips ... noticing there may be tingling, there may be warmth, just noticing whatever you feel ... *Pause for fifteen seconds.* Now, bring your awareness to your left shoulder, allowing awareness to move gradually down your left arm, the upper arm and tricep, the left elbow, the left forearm, wrist. Feel the back of your let hand, feeling the palm of your left hand, and feeling your left fingers, allowing sensation to reach into your left fingertips, just gently noticing every sensation without judging, gently guiding your mind back when you've noticed that it has wandered. *Pause for ten seconds.* Now, move your attention to your neck and your throat, feeling the muscles in the back of your neck, feeling the tender vulnerable area of the front of your throat, noticing if there is any sensation, any tension, and letting your awareness travel up the back of your neck to your scalp and the back of your head. Feel your ears, and then move your attention forward to notice your jaw. Just notice if any tension is held there. *Pause for ten seconds.* Bring attention now to your chin, and notice the sensations in your lips, noticing the inside of your mouth, your tongue, your teeth and your gums, the inside of your throat, now bringing attention to your nose and your cheekbones. *Pause for ten seconds.* Bring attention to your eyes, noticing the many tiny muscles surrounding your eyes, just noticing all the many sensations, the feeling of your eyeballs inside your eye sockets, the feeling of your eyebrows, and then bring attention to your forehead, and finally bringing attention to the crown of your head, noticing any sensations of energy at the top of your body. *Pause for five seconds.* Now, see if you can bring awareness to your entire body at once. *Pause for fifteen seconds.* At this point, you may not feel any sensation or you may feel sensation. Can you experience the field of energy that is your body? Can you rest in that awareness of your whole energy field? If you'd like, you can imagine that as your breathe in, the breath enters your body through the crown of your head and sweeps through your body, and as you exhale, the breath exits through your feet. In this way you can imagine that you're floating on a gentle wave of breath, gently moving in and out of your body, holding you. *Pause for fifteen seconds.* Now, continue to rest in this posture for the next several minutes. Focus on your nose, and feel the air as it enters your nose ... then feel the air as it departs out of your nose. *Pause for ten seconds.* If you feel your mind wandering, gently bring your attention back to your nose, focusing on the sensations that come with the air entering and exiting through your nose. Allow your body to release ... Just let it all go ...

We hope you have found this mindfulness exercise to be effective in reducing your tension and helping to increase your focus. As you return to your normal activities, remember that mindfulness is a skill you can continually work toward improving. When the urge strikes, when you are alone or perhaps in conversation with others, challenge yourself to be more mindful and allow yourself to be actively involved in and aware of your surroundings. You'll find that increased mindfulness has many benefits for your mental health and the quality of your relationships with other people.

SELF-HYPNOSIS TRAINING

The final strategy presented in this chapter that can be useful toward managing your anxiety, depression, and pain symptoms is learning how to do self-hypnosis. *Hypnosis* is a naturally occurring state of mind that can be defined as a heightened state of focused concentration (trance) and a willingness to follow instructions and that often involves increased suggestibility. Hypnosis can successfully be used to address undesirable habits such as smoking and overeating; emotional issues such as depression, anxiety, and low self-esteem; some medical issues such as pain; and other goals that might include improving your study skills or occupational or recreational performance. When the heightened state of concentration and increased focus is induced without the assistance of a therapist or hypnotist, this process is referred to as *self-hypnosis*.

Self-hypnosis is widely used today, and it differs from the traditional notion of hypnosis in that it not only does not require a hypnotist, but it also involves developing a state of relaxation that is deep but in a conscious state, as opposed to the unconscious state often induced by a hypnotist. Self-hypnosis can be used in a variety of ways that may be useful for someone across all stages of cancer, ranging from the reduction of anticipatory stress that might be associated with meeting with doctors or undergoing a particular cancer treatment to the reduction of the experience of physical pain to the elimination of many psychological symptoms that would include anxiety and depression.

A similar approach to self-hypnosis therapy is referred to as *autogenic therapy*, which was developed in the twentieth century by Dr. Johannes Schultz, a psychiatrist and neurologist. Autogenic therapy is used to produce deep relaxation and promote the reduction of stress, often using self-commands aimed at producing relaxation through developing better body control, including regulating breathing, heart rate, blood pressure, and temperature. Autogenic therapy is focused on the creation of a feeling of warmth and heaviness throughout the body, thereby providing the experience of a profound state of physical relaxation, bodily health, and mental peace. The aim of autogenic training is to change a state of arousal associated with sympathetic activity of the autonomic nervous system to one of profound relaxation associated with the parasympathetic system (recall these terms from chapter 3). In training yourself in autogenic procedures, you learn to become a passive observer in an altered state of consciousness, a relaxed state believed to be helpful in promoting psychological well-being. Although autogenic therapy is a unique approach in some ways, its shares many features with the process of self-hypnosis. Therefore, we will consider both approaches together as hypnosis-based approaches through the remainder of this section.

Effectiveness of Hypnosis-Based Approaches

Hypnosis-based approaches have increasingly gained support as effective strategies to address issues of depression, anxiety, and pain. This next section focuses on some of the supporting evidence for these strategies and helps you determine whether self-hypnosis might be an effective strategy for you to learn and incorporate into your daily routine.

A GOOD STRATEGY FOR PAIN

An independent panel from the National Institutes of Health concluded that there was strong evidence for the use of hypnosis in alleviating chronic pain associated with cancer (NIMH 1995). As a basis for this conclusion, a number of important research studies have pointed to the benefits of hypnosis in acute and chronic pain and cancer pain. For example, Spiegel and Bloom (1983) examined pain control and other variables in women with chronic cancer pain associated with breast carcinoma. In this study, fifty-four women were assigned to either a usual treatment control condition (twenty-four women) or to a group receiving usual treatment and weekly group therapy for up to twelve months (thirty women). The women in group therapy were, in turn, assigned to groups that either did or did not have brief (five- to ten-minute) self-hypnosis as a part of their group therapy treatment. Both support groups showed improvement in pain control compared with patients in usual treatment. However, women who received self-hypnosis showed an additional improvement in pain intensity compared with the cancer patients receiving group therapy without self-hypnosis.

In a second study (Syrjala et al. 1995) bone marrow transplant patients with oral pain were assigned to one of four treatment conditions: treatment as usual; therapist support, which included an educational component and reassurance but not the training of new coping skills; relaxation/imagery/autogenic training; and a cognitive-behavioral skills-training program. Results revealed that patients in the relaxation/imagery/autogenic training group and the cognitive-behavioral skills group reported significantly less pain than those in the treatment-as-usual group.

Finally, a third study was aimed at determining the impact of brief presurgical hypnosis on patients' postsurgery pain and distress (Montgomery et al. 2002). In this study, twenty breast biopsy patients were assigned to either a hypnosis group or a control group (treatment as usual). Hypnosis was found to significantly reduce postsurgery pain and distress. A number of other comprehensive reviews have supported the use of hypnosis in acute and chronic pain and cancer pain (Hawkins 2001; Montgomery, DuHamel, and Redd 2000; Patterson and Jensen 2003).

A GOOD STRATEGY FOR ENHANCING THE IMMUNE RESPONSE

In addition to reducing symptoms of pain, there is evidence to suggest that hypnosis can effectively modify the production and activity of components of the immune system and the immune-system response as measured by B-cells, T-cells, and helper cells and suppressor cells (Gruzelier 2002). The principal function of these types of cells is to make antibodies that can assist the body in fighting off disease and illness, making them essential toward having an adaptive and highly functioning immune system. Such immune-system control is often accompanied by self-reports of enhanced mood and psychological well-being. Some studies have even suggested that this immune-system enhancement in cancer patients may translate into longer survival time, although further studies are required to confirm these findings (Walker, Heys, and Eremin 1999).

Several recent studies by John Gruzelier and his colleagues have explored the impact of self-hypnosis on the immune system (Gruzelier, Smith et al. 2001; Gruzelier, Levy et al. 2001; Gruzelier et al. 2002). In two studies, hypnosis reduced the effects of stress on immune functioning in medical students at exam time. The implications for health were investigated in a third study in patients with a chronic herpes simplex virus (HSV-2). Six weeks of self-hypnosis training reduced the recurrence of outbreaks and reduced levels of clinical depression and anxiety. Immune functions were greatly improved, most notably functional natural killer cell activity. In a study more directly related to cancer patients, Spiegel and colleagues (1989) carried out a ten-year follow-up of eighty-six women with metastatic breast cancer, some of whom received group therapy consisting of a variety of interventions including peer-group support, emotional expression, relaxation training, and self-hypnosis. The mean survival time of patients receiving group therapy was 36.6 months compared with 18.9 months in the control group. The precise mechanism involved with the intervention enhancing survival time in this study is somewhat unclear. The investigators suggested that the intervention may have enhanced compliance with medical treatment, improved appetite and nutritional intake, and enabled patients to maintain an increased level of healthy physical activity.

More recently, a trial of relaxation training and guided imagery in eighty women with large or locally advanced breast cancer was carried out to assess the effects of this intervention on host defenses in patients with cancer. In addition to improving quality of life (Walker et al. 1999), the intervention increased the number and percentage of activated T cells. This and the previous study point to the conclusion that cancer patients receiving treatments such as self-hypnosis, relaxation, and imagery training can produce immunological changes and more positive mental health.

A GOOD STRATEGY FOR REDUCING NEGATIVE MOODS

As you are already aware, many cancer patients may experience stress, anxiety, and often depression. Such negative mood states are also associated with a depressed natural defense system, both from the disease itself and from its treatment (Spiegel and Giese-Davis 2003; Walker et al. 1997). Consequently, researchers have begun to examine the effects of self-hypnosis autogenic training on mood and anxiety as well. In general, results have been encouraging.

For instance, Wright, Courtney, and Crowther (2002) examined the effectiveness of a ten-week autogenic training as a complementary therapy for patients with cancer, with the aim of increasing their coping abilities. Findings revealed a significant reduction in anxiety and increase in "fighting spirit" relative to pretreatment, with additional improvements in the ability to cope and have a more efficient night's sleep. Lyles and colleagues (1982) assigned fifty cancer patients receiving chemotherapy to one of three conditions: progressive muscle relaxation training plus guided relaxation imagery; therapist support, in which a therapist provided support and encouragement but not relaxation training; and a no-treatment control group. Results indicated that patients who received relaxation and imagery training reported feeling significantly less anxious and nauseated during chemotherapy, showed significantly less physiological arousal (as measured by pulse rate and systolic blood pressure), reported less anxiety and depression immediately after chemotherapy; and reported significantly less severe nausea at home following chemotherapy.

Liossi and White (2001) evaluated the efficacy of clinical hypnosis in the enhancement of quality of life of patients with advanced cancer. Fifty terminally ill cancer patients received either routine medical and psychological care or standard care plus hypnosis. Patients in the hypnosis group received weekly sessions of hypnosis with a therapist for four weeks. Results demonstrated that at the end of the intervention period, patients in the hypnosis group had significantly higher self-reported quality of life and lower levels of anxiety and depression compared to the standard care group.

In another recent study, Laidlaw and Willett (2002) assigned thirty-five cancer patients suffering from acute anxiety attacks to receive a tape teaching either progressive muscular relaxation or a light and slow breathing rhythm, both delivered in the context of hypnosis. Participants showed significant improvement as measured by both reduced frequency of acute anxiety episodes and decreased self-reported depression and anxiety.

Despite the encouraging findings we've seen here, it's important to mention that results are not always positive, and there are currently too few controlled studies to make definitive statements about the role of hypnosis-based approaches for cancer patients. Further, even when effective, the exact mechanism through which these approaches may work also is unclear at present. However, we propose that there currently is enough support for self-hypnosis-based interventions that it is useful to present this strategy to you as a potential tool that might be incorporated into your life to help you overcome your depression, anxiety, and pain symptoms.

Are Hypnosis-Based Approaches Right for You?

It's important to recognize that like most things in life, hypnosis-based approaches are unlikely to work if they are not practiced regularly. Therefore, it is crucial to make a commitment to setting aside a time each day when you can learn to develop this skill. Just as with progressive muscle relaxation and mindfulness training, a key to success is limiting potential distractions (for instance, lower the volume on your telephone or turn off your cell phone, practice when you are home alone). Further, it has been suggested that one should avoid eating, smoking, or drinking before practice, as the digestive processes may interfere with the effectiveness of hypnotic procedures. Although hypnosis-based approaches are largely considered safe and generally should not be feared, individuals with abnormal blood pressure, diabetes, or a serious heart condition should consult with a physician before beginning this type of therapy.

Hypnosis can give you a greater ability to be in control of yourself. In making the decision to learn hypnosis, you are making a commitment to practice skills that allow you to better use the abilities that you already possess. The possibilities of hypnosis are substantial. As alluded to earlier, you can help your body achieve greater comfort and a sense of well-being, lessen or remove pain, improve immune system functioning, improve your performance in various areas of your life, overcome anxiety, fear, and depression, and generally increase your focus and concentration.

In deciding whether or not self-hypnosis may be a useful approach for you to use, consider that the more of these characteristics apply to you, the greater the likelihood you might benefit:

You generally are not opposed to hypnosis and believe it is possible to be hypnotized.

You are open to new experiences.

You are comfortable with letting yourself relax and letting go.

You are capable of being imaginative.

You are a good listener.

You are motivated to change your behaviors and emotional experiences, whether it is depression, anxiety, pain, or some activity or behavior.

Self-hypnosis instructions. Self-hypnosis can be beneficial for many people, and many different hypnotic strategies and induction techniques are available to be tried. For the following exercise, we chose an induction strategy by Charles Henderson (2007) that might be particularly useful for you to practice and incorporate into your life. It might be most useful for you to record the instructions to use on a daily basis. As you make the recording, try to speak normally, but also try to make sure you speak at a relatively slow pace and with as soothing a voice as possible. When you engage in self-hypnosis, remember to be patient and just allow yourself the freedom to let go of your surroundings and focus on the instructions on the recording. Do not try to force yourself to be hypnotized—just try to let it happen. Hypnosis is a very different experience for each person who tries it, but remember that it is always a pleasant experience that is very soothing, and you will get better at it as you practice.

For the following exercise, get into a comfortable position. Most people prefer to practice while lying down. Concentrate without any goal, and use your visual imagination and verbal cues to relax your body as much as possible. The exercise will take between ten and twenty minutes.

"I am starting my self-hypnosis session now. From now until I say 'wake up' I will get more and more relaxed and focused within myself. Suggestions I give myself will be effective, but this will apply to only those suggestions I consciously want to be effective.

As I close my eyes and begin to drift downward, I can imagine a blanket covering my feet. Every part of my body covered by the blanket will become completely relaxed. My feet are becoming deeply relaxed. All of the muscles in my feet are becoming limp and relaxed.

Now the blanket is moving up to my knees. Every muscle and tendon in my body from my knees down is getting more and more relaxed. All the tension is flowing out of this area, leaving all the muscles limp and loose.

Now the blanket is moving slowly up to my waist. As it moves upward, everything is becoming relaxed. As it reaches my waist, I can hardly feel anything from there on down. All the muscles in my hips, lower abdomen, legs, and feet are becoming progressively more and more relaxed.

All cares are flowing out of my mind. If a thought does intrude I will just gently let it go away. I am thinking only of relaxing and letting go of all tension. All of my muscles are becoming more and more relaxed, and I am feeling pleasantly drowsy. I will not go to sleep, but I am feeling so carefree and relaxed, sinking further and further into myself with no cares or worries.

Now the blanket is moving upward, moving slowly over my stomach, inching up over my chest, stopping at my shoulders. All of the muscles in my stomach and back are letting go, becoming totally and completely relaxed. The relaxation is like a warmness, spreading to every place covered by the blanket. The muscles in my chest and arms are getting more and more limp. I could move if I really had to, but I am becoming so comfortably limp and relaxed that I really don't want to move. I am still and relaxed, drifting deeper and deeper into a pleasant state of dreamy relaxation.

Now the warmth and relaxation are slowly moving upward from my shoulders. The blanket is remaining there, but the relaxation is gently moving upward into my neck. All the muscles in my neck are becoming limp and flaccid. In my mind's eye, I can see them becoming limp and loose. All cares and worries are floating away as I drift deeper and deeper into my relaxation.

Now the relaxation is spreading into my mouth and jaw muscles. My tongue is limp, resting in my mouth with no need to be tense. I may briefly have more saliva in my mouth, but that will go away shortly. Now my cheeks and eyes are relaxing. I could open my eyes if I wanted to, but unless I need to, it would be too much work. It would take too much effort to open my eyes. I am drifting pleasantly downward, becoming more and more relaxed.

The muscles in my forehead are becoming more and more relaxed. I can imagine them, like rubber bands across my forehead, becoming limp and floppy. Deeper and deeper, relaxing more and more. From the tips of my toes to the top of my head, I am becoming more and more relaxed, drifting downward, deeper and deeper.

Now I am going to count down from twenty-five. As I count down I will continue to drift down, pleasantly going deeper and deeper into the relaxation. I will get drowsy and deeply relaxed, but I will not actually go to sleep. I will simply drift deeper and deeper into my self-hypnotic state of deeply relaxed awareness. By the time I reach zero I will be in a very pleasant, sleeplike state. I will still be able to direct my thoughts, and I could rouse myself immediately if I needed to, but unless I really need to, I will drift deeper and deeper into the relaxation.

Starting down now ... twenty-five ... twenty-four ... twenty-three ... twenty-two ... drifting deeper and deeper with each count ... twenty-one ... twenty ... feeling drowsier and drowsier, yet still awake ... nineteen ... eighteen ... seventeen ... floating gently downward with each count ... sixteen ... fifteen ... fourteen ... drifting, drowsy ... thirteen ... twelve ... eleven ... ten ... more than halfway down, drifting deeper and deeper with each count ... nine ... eight ... seven ... six ... five ... feeling so relaxed ... four ... becoming more and more relaxed and drowsy ... three ... two ... one ... zero ... breathing pleasantly, slowly, drifting deeper and deeper with each breath.

As I continue to be deeply relaxed, and to become even more relaxed, I am thinking about what I want to change about myself. [*Something like the following may be useful, but you will want to make this section as specific to your problems as possible*] I will change the way I am spending my time during the day. There are so many opportunities for me to find more pleasure in my life, and I am going to start taking advantage of these opportunities. I am going to start interacting with people more often. I am going to be more active when it comes to participating in activities that would make me happy. I am going to be an active person in this world and make good use of my time. I will find happiness and pleasure, and I will face things that cause me to feel anxiety. I will not avoid places, people, or things that cause me discomfort. I am fully capable of meeting my fears and anxieties head on. I need to face these situations so that I will overcome my fears and anxieties … so I can be happier in my life. I will not allow pain to slow me down. Pain will come and go in my life, but I can cope with pain when I experience it, and I can still continue to do the things I need to do in my life to make me a happier, more fulfilled person. I owe it to myself to be happier, and I am fully capable of becoming a more positive person. I am not going to let anything stand in the way of my journey toward happiness. I will not let my fear and anxiety stand in the way. I will not let pain stand in the way. I am going to change the way I behave, I am going to be more active, and I am going to become an improved person.

All of these suggestions that I have given myself will be effective because they are right for me and it is good that I should achieve them. All of the directions I have given myself are good for me and I will follow them.

Each time I practice self-hypnosis I will become better and better at it. I will be able to relax deeper and deeper in less time with each practice.

Now, as I count to three, I am going to slowly, gradually, pleasantly become more alert from my relaxed state. I will return to my normal, waking state, except for the suggested changes. Now, starting to become a little more alert … one … becoming more alert … two … getting ready to wake up … three, completely alert."

As you practice the exercises we have presented in this chapter, we hope that you will experience many benefits in your ability to relax, feel less depressed, and experience less pain. This concludes the behavioral-activation and skill-building component of this workbook and leaves one final but very central issue that will be critical if you are to optimally benefit from the methods you've learned here. Specifically, now that you have the tools you need to overcome feelings of depression and anxiety, you need a plan to ensure that you continue to recall these skills and incorporate them as part of your regular activities. The issue of maintaining these skills and preventing a relapse into depression and anxiety is the focus of the final chapter.

CHAPTER 11

Maintaining Treatment Gains and Preventing Relapse

TIME: Approximately One Week, Then Reviewed as Needed

As you have progressed through this book, you have had the chance to develop a wide range of skills to help you use behavioral activation to overcome feelings of anxiety and depression associated with your cancer diagnosis. Although this is the final chapter, it is only the beginning in your battle against cancer and the anxiety and depression that may accompany it. Just as you need to pay attention to your cancer, even if it is in remission, the same level of focus is needed to stay psychologically healthy and prevent a relapse back to feeling heightened levels of anxiety and depression. In this case, that means paying attention to your psychological health at all times, including the times when you feel good. This isn't to say you should become overly concerned to the extent that you spend a large portion of your time worrying about falling back into a troublesome state of depression or anxiety. However, giving a little attention to your emotional experiences will go a long way. This is especially true given that research indicates that relapse is a real risk among people who have experienced depression. The risk of relapse after one episode of major depression is 50 percent, and after two episodes it is 80 percent (Katon et al. 2001). We don't present these high rates to suggest that you're doomed to once again feel those problematic feelings of depression or anxiety, but instead to suggest the importance of preparing for the possibility that it might happen, regardless of how positive you may feel right now. So, if the bad news is that relapse is a real phenomenon, then the good news is that, as real as it is, it can also be prevented. In fact, one of the most highly supported methods for preventing relapse is the continued use of treatment strategies, from medication all the way through self-directed manuals such as the one you have just experienced. Given these realities, we will turn to clear and practical strategies to stay psychologically healthy and prevent a relapse back to the feelings of depression and anxiety that led you to this book in the first place.

RECOGNIZING HOW FAR YOU'VE COME

When you first began the journey through this self-help workbook, you were experiencing problems with depression and anxiety. As you reflect on where you were when you began this workbook, and where you are right now, what have you learned about yourself? How have you changed? Use the space below to write down your thoughts.

EXERCISE: YOUR PROGRESS

Think about the changes you have made in your life and how differently you are behaving now compared to when you began this workbook. How have these behavioral changes affected your mood?

_____

_____

_____

_____

_____

_____

_____

Although we are aware that behavioral-activation strategies presented in this workbook help a substantial number of people, we also recognize that not everyone benefits to the same degree. As you think about your experiences, how beneficial have the strategies been toward reducing your symptoms of depression and anxiety? (Circle one.)

1	2	3	4	5
(Not helpful		Somewhat helpful		Extremely helpful)

As you think about this rating, consider why you responded the way that you did. What did you find most helpful about this workbook? What was least helpful?

_____

_____

_____

_____

_____

THE IMPORTANCE OF CONTINUED ASSESSMENT

A key component toward your success with preventing a relapse back to depression and anxiety is that of continued self-assessment. At this point you are probably very used to being assessed by someone else, from physicians, oncologists, nurses, and other medical staff who have helped you work through your cancer to possibly mental health professionals such as psychiatrists, psychologists, or social workers for your state of mind and psychological well being. However, when it comes to staying on top of your recovery and continuing to use the skills taught in this book, the role of continued self-assessment cannot be overemphasized.

What do we mean by self-assessment? Well, this could mean a lot of different things for different situations and different people. In general, it means always taking some time to be aware of how you are doing and taking steps to address potential problems before they begin to seem tremendously overwhelming. This might sound simple, especially after all the effort you have put toward your recovery. Further, the behavioral-activation strategies you have begun to utilize in this manual have been about planning ahead and improving how you feel through taking active steps toward achieving your values and goals. However, it can sometimes be hard to keep up with this daily process of behavioral activation, especially if you have dramatically changed how you spend your time during the day and are working toward engaging in multiple behaviors. Quite interestingly, this may especially become a concern once you start feeling better. Indeed, as the strategies start to work and you begin to move forward with your life, it isn't reasonable to expect you to devote the level of time and effort to your recovery from anxiety and depression as you likely have done up to this point. With that being the case, the strategies are unlikely to continue to work and you are unlikely to continue to feel psychologically healthy without some attention to these issues.

Most people are aware that major traumatic events (such as the reemergence of cancer, loss of a loved one, loss of a job) can lead one back to feelings of anxiety and depression, but small everyday issues are much more likely to be what sets you back in your progress. The good news is that with some attention, these small issues can be addressed before they snowball into a major episode of depression or anxiety. Indeed, the secret to preventing relapse is not struggling to pull yourself up when you start to feel really badly and get to the lowest of lows but instead learning to get back on track when you begin to feel badly.

To illustrate this point, let's consider an example. Imagine that someone was willing to give you your dream house for free. The only catch is that the plumbing is a little old and there are a few valves that on occasion will become loose and require simple tightening. If a loose valve was identified within a day or so of it becoming loose, it could be easily tightened with no problem. However, if it was left loose for a few days, then a leak might develop, with a full-blown flood likely to follow soon after. The generous benefactor who is giving you the house summarizes the situation in the following way: "Basically, you could live in your dream house for free for the rest of your life, but you would have to do a brief status check every morning and evening to make sure that the valves are tight. If they are, then everything is great and you can go on with your life. If they aren't tight, you can stop for a few moments, tighten any that are loose, and then everything will be great and you can go on with your life." He also provides a word of caution. The last owner was very diligent when she first moved in, checking the valves repeatedly throughout the day. The valves were rarely loose, and after some time, she began checking them less and less. But the more time that went by, the looser the valves got, until one day, after the valves weren't checked for a very lengthy period of time, a valve burst and caused a very costly flood.

The purpose of this example is to make the point that you have put a lot of work into overcoming depression and anxiety associated with your cancer diagnosis. At first you may have rapidly moved through this book and the exercises in it. This initial burst of energy probably was very useful in helping you to travel down the right track to psychological health. Unfortunately, your recovery is not a job to be *completed*, but a lifelong journey to psychological health accompanied by your journey toward physical health. So, if it is human nature to begin to lose steam once you start to feel better, how do you stay aware of the possibility of becoming depressed or anxious while also staying positive and enjoying your success? Part of this process involves the movement toward being proactive and movement away from being reactive, an important distinction we turn to next.

Proactive vs. Reactive Strategies to Prevent Relapse

Starting with their definitions, *proactive* refers to acting in anticipation of future problems, needs, or changes, while *reactive* refers to acting in response to a problem and/or the stress or emotional upset resulting from that problem. Especially as we become busy in our lives, it becomes easy to fall into the trap of addressing problems in a reactive manner. Stated differently, we often address problems as they happen instead of before they happen. This strategy then becomes a vicious cycle because new fires develop while we are busy trying to put out the old ones. This problem is compounded by the fact that some people become so good at putting out fires when they happen that they stop trying to prevent them in the first place. Although this might work at first, it often becomes too exhausting over time, and there end up being more fires than any one person could hope to put out. At this point, anxiety and depression are natural consequences.

The first question to ask is why it is so tempting to slip back to being reactive. We argue that one primary reason is that it's hard to get yourself to stop and identify potential problems, especially when you're feeling good. In fact, some may worry that this approach means that you are doubting yourself or worrying when there is no reason to do so. In fact, the condition of generalized anxiety disorder involves a continued state of worry where someone overthinks what can go wrong and becomes paralyzed with fear about these issues. Alternatively, it might even feel like this is simply focusing on the negatives. We understand this sentiment, but we also believe that honestly coming to understand your vulnerability to the possible pitfalls ahead of you can help you to be more equipped to handle them if they do happen.

To illustrate the point, imagine you are a parent with a teenage daughter who has asked to go to a party on Friday night. You pause for a second and then start to ask questions that will help you assess the safety of the situation and plan how to handle the situation if you decide to give permission. For instance, you might ask if parents will be home, if the kids will be drinking, how your daughter will get home, what time she is planning to get there, and what time she is planning to come home. You believe these are all reasonable questions, but before you even have a chance to say a word, she groans and storms up the stairs complaining that if you can't just say yes, then you must not trust her. Being a super parent, you head up to her room and sit down on the bed next to her. You begin by saying that of course you trust her, but that isn't the issue. The issue is that in all situations there is some risk, so it's important to gather information to determine that risk and then plan accordingly. After she calms down, you begin your assessment by asking questions. Following her answers, you suggest that the two of you consider things that could go wrong and develop a proactive plan. She tells you that she is getting a ride from a friend and that she is certain there won't be alcohol or drugs at the party. A reactive approach would stop the planning at that, leaving her stuck to come up with a solution if something were to suddenly go wrong. Instead, you take a proactive approach and suggest that you both brainstorm what she will do if alcohol appears at the party, including how your daughter will get home (especially if her friend who is driving decides to drink). The point that you try to reinforce is that you aren't dwelling on the negative, expecting something to necessarily go wrong, and certainly not suggesting that you mistrust her, but more that you want her to be prepared if something does go wrong.

Taking the example above, we would like you to identify situations that might present a risk for your relapse back to anxiety and depression. To help with this goal, let's walk through several examples together, one specific to anxiety regarding the possible return of cancer, a second related to adjustment once cancer is no longer the primary focus of your life, and a third that's not related to cancer at all, but may be likely to lead to anxiety and depression that certainly can affect your physical health. For each example, follow along with the items entered into the corresponding table. When you are finished going through these examples, try and create a scenario of your own in the attached form.

EXAMPLE 1: AVOIDING THE CHECKUP

Let's imagine a situation in which you have to go to your oncologist for a regular check-up six months after the remission of your cancer. For three weeks prior to the appointment you notice you have begun to ruminate about what might happen at the appointment. You just ignore these feelings, and then on the day you are supposed to go to the doctor's office, you start to feel so sick that you can't even leave the house. You don't call the doctor to cancel but just go into your room, shut the door, crawl into bed, and lie down. Although this strategy presents initial relief, you quickly begin to ruminate about the consequences of your decision, and soon the worry has spiraled out of control to the point where you feel as if you are losing touch with your life and you feel your health is being compromised.

EXAMPLE 2: TRANSITIONING TO REMISSION

Now imagine a situation in which you have aggressively begun to treat your cancer. These efforts take over your life and become the focus of almost every waking moment between chemotherapy and other medical-related activities. At the same time you notice feeling anxious, depressed, and angry. To help address these issues, you begin the strategies outlined here to address your psychological well being. Thanks to effective treatment, you cancer goes into remission, and because of your hard work, you find yourself feeling as psychologically healthy as you ever have felt. Because these efforts are exhausting, you take the next few weeks to slow down, unwind, and give yourself a chance to breathe. After a few weeks, however, you start to notice that the feeling of relaxation now seems to be replaced by a feeling of uncertainty and, in a strange way, a loss of purpose. Being reactive might include ignoring these feelings until they mushroom into another round of full-blown anxiety and depressive symptoms. In contrast, a proactive approach might involve talking to someone about what you are feeling, as well as resuming your behavioral activation exercises to be sure to keep your focus on valued goals and to restore the activity and purpose you felt while you were struggling to get healthy.

EXAMPLE 3: REACHING OUT

Imagine you are quite busy and have begun to lose touch with a friend. Taking a reactive approach, you might let the relationship slip until it gets to the point where your friend might call you to tell you that she feels very hurt that you have disappeared from her life, at which point you feel awful and suggest several immediate strategies to try to fix the situation. In contrast, a proactive approach would require you to stop and recognize that this friendship is important to you and that you need to reach out to her now, before she gets hurt and disappointed. Of course, because you are very busy, you may not have a lot of time to spend with this person. But simply reaching out to this friend has shown that you care and will enable you to stop worrying about it in the back of your mind at all times.

PROACTIVE STRATEGIES WORKSHEET: EXAMPLE

Situation	Proactive Strategies
Describe the situation: *Having to go back to the doctor to have a check-up following remission* **Key issues:** ■ *I know someone whose cancer came back.* ■ *I don't want to talk about my worries with others now that I'm better.* ■ *I don't know if I have the energy to fight my cancer the way I did last time.*	**Assess the situation:** ■ *I am worried I might get bad news from the oncologist.* ■ *I also have more general feelings of anxiety and nervousness.* ■ *I am lonely, and there is no one I trust that I can talk to about my fears.* ■ *I think I might feel nauseous when I arrive at the oncologist's office.* **Take proactive steps:** ■ *Identify what can you do now and in the time before the appointment to help you on that day, especially if you get nervous.* ■ *Get a support person to come with you to the appointment.* ■ *Expect good news but prepare for what you will do if you get bad news so that you will not be caught off guard.* ■ *Speak to a physician or counselor about receiving treatment for these feelings.*

PROACTIVE STRATEGIES WORKSHEET

Situation	Proactive Strategies
Describe the situation: **Key issues:**	**Assess the situation:** **Take proactive steps:**

MINDING THE STORE: CONTINUED ASSESSMENT AND PRACTICE

The primary goal of this chapter is to point out that as you move forward in your life past cancer and the anxiety and depression that have come along with it, it is important to stay focused on both your physical and psychological health through ongoing assessment and the use of proactive as opposed to reactive strategies. In doing so, some people may find it helpful to use the full behavioral-activation program outlined in this workbook. However, others may find it more difficult to continue with the structure the program provides on a daily basis. For this reason, we conclude with a modified version of the treatment that can be used for a few minutes twice a day to help you stay focused with minimal investment. Because this is something we believe you might benefit from for the rest of your life, we will refer to it as the *maintenance program*.

This maintenance program includes an opportunity to reflect, on a daily basis at the start of each day, on four questions to keep you on track in your recovery, including: (1) What would you like to accomplish today? (2) What are things you have to look forward to today to stay positive? (3) What are the proactive steps you need to take today? and (4) What are the supports you can rely on today to achieve your goals, stay positive, and take necessary proactive steps? This is then followed with a similar set of questions in the evening that help you reflect on the extent to which you lived your day in the way you had hoped when it started. In taking just a few minutes each day to complete this brief check-in, you will be able to stay focused on what's important to you and evaluate your success in achieving these goals. If you find that you are setting reasonable goals in the morning and achieving them by day's end most of the time, then you will have good reason to be confident about your ability to stay psychologically healthy. However, this also can be helpful to indicate the source of problems if things aren't going well. For instance, if you're finding that you can't meet your goals for the day and are slipping back into negative feelings, think about whether the problem is that you are setting your goals too high or if it is that you're simply having trouble completing reasonable goals. In either case, you might consider returning to the full behavioral-activation program presented in this workbook to go through the steps of determining values and goals and setting yourself up with the structure you need to achieve these goals. In fact, in keeping with the idea of life as a journey as opposed to a destination, you might find yourself coming back to the full program at different times in your life and only using the more brief maintenance format at other times, depending on what your particular needs are at a particular time. Always remember that if you do have to return to the program, this does not mean that you have failed in any way. Everyone has certain experiences in their lives where they lose contact with pleasurable or rewarding experiences, events, or behaviors. This happens because we live in a changing world where the people we interact with, our home life, circumstances at work, and opportunities to engage in various activities and hobbies are ever changing. So if you find yourself becoming depressed or anxious somewhere down the road, think of it as a problem with your environment and changes in your life that have resulted in decreased opportunities to have pleasurable or positive experiences. Then recognize this experience as a need to get back to what you have learned, namely behavioral activation.

Next, we present the two maintenance forms (morning and evening), including a sample and one set for you to copy and complete on your own. We recommend making copies for a full week at the start of the week and keeping them in a place where you can easily access them and spend a few minutes each morning and evening completing them.

DAILY ASSESSMENT PLANNER (MORNING)   Date: _____

What would I like to accomplish today? *Today I would like to go through my bills that have been sitting in a box. I also would like to make a healthy dinner for the family and have some nice conversation at dinner. I need to call my sister and begin to make plans for Thanksgiving. Finally, I would like to take my full lunch hour at work. In addition to eating slowly and enjoying my food, I also can take some time to practice my breathing exercises.*

What are things I have to look forward to today to stay positive today? *I'm looking forward to spending some time with my children tonight. I have been so busy that it seems like I don't really get to talk with them anymore. I am going to make their favorite dinner and I've planned some things to talk about at dinner to keep conversation going. Most of all, I look forward to having some relaxing time with them and seeing them smile.*

Are there any proactive steps I need to take today? *In addition to preparing for the things I listed above, I also need to set up a meeting with my boss. Ever since I came back to work, I feel like I haven't been given the same level of responsibility. I want to tell him how I feel and see if there is anything I can do differently to help smooth my transition back at work. I have been worrying about this every night, which is effecting my sleep, so I need to at least set up the meeting today.*

What are the supports I can rely on today? *Knowing I will get to see my kids tonight will be a great support that I can look forward to throughout the day. I also know my sister is always there for me, so if I get stuck on any of my goals today, I might call her and problem solve for a few minutes. I also can chat with her for a few minutes about how her day is going, as she is going through some tough times now.*

DAILY ASSESSMENT PLANNER (EVENING)   Date: _____

What did I accomplish today and what about the things I did not accomplish today? *I went through my bills and organized them. I need to pay them another day, but this was a good start and will make paying them easier. I did prepare dinner, and I had my conversation topics all ready. I did have to cut lunch short today because of an unexpected deadline, so I will need to be sure to prioritize that tomorrow.*

What did I enjoy today? *I am in such a good mood after dinner. The kids had a lot to say, and I didn't even use my conversation topics—but I was glad I had them, just in case. The food was great, and they really appreciated me making their favorite dish. They almost didn't notice the vegetables that came with it. Having something like this to look forward to would sure help get through the tough times now that I'm back at work.*

Did I take the proactive steps I needed to today? If not, what happened? *I was so busy at work today that I didn't even remember to set up a meeting with my boss. I am feeling great tonight, so I probably won't have trouble sleeping because of it. But I can't just forget about it because it will affect me sooner or later. I will put it in my planner for tomorrow so when I see it, it will be my cue to go and arrange the meeting.*

What supports helped today, and what other supports are needed? *Looking forward to seeing the kids really did help like I thought it would, especially when I had to cut lunch short. I also had a great conversation with my sister. It was very short, but I made sure I carved out five minutes to speak to her. I think she really appreciated me taking the time out for her, as well. After all she has been doing for me, it felt really nice to be able to show her some support.*

DAILY ASSESSMENT PLANNER (MORNING)   Date: _____

What would I like to accomplish today?

_____

_____

_____

_____

What are things I have to look forward to today to stay positive today?

_____

_____

_____

_____

Are there any proactive steps I need to take today?

_____

_____

_____

_____

What are the supports I can rely on today?

_____

_____

_____

_____

DAILY ASSESSMENT PLANNER (EVENING)   Date: _____

What did I accomplish today and what about the things I did not accomplish today?

_____

_____

_____

_____

_____

What did I enjoy today?

_____

_____

_____

_____

Did I take the proactive steps I needed to today? If not, what happened?

_____

_____

_____

_____

What supports helped today and what other supports are needed?

_____

_____

_____

_____

DIFFERENT TREATMENT OPTIONS

Although we are optimistic and hopeful that the behavioral-activation treatment and supplemental strategies we've offered in this workbook have effectively assisted you in overcoming your depression and anxiety, we also recognize that no treatment works for everyone. Therefore, if you are still experiencing fairly troublesome symptoms of depression or anxiety, you may want to consider some different strategies.

As addressed in the introduction of this book, treatment options for major depression generally include psychotherapeutic, pharmacological, and alternative approaches. Much like the behavioral activation strategies presented in this book, other psychological therapy approaches work on teaching you skills to behave differently to improve or decrease your symptoms. For example, *cognitive therapy* was developed to more specifically examine the way you think about life events and situations and how the specific thoughts you have about situations or experiences might sometimes be irrational or maladaptive and contribute to symptoms of anxiety and depression (Beck et al. 1979). *Interpersonal psychotherapy* is based on the notion that problems with interpersonal relationships and your social roles and behaviors are linked with depression, and treatment strategies are designed to increase your awareness of social-role changes, address interpersonal disputes and conflicts, overcome social-skill deficits, and process any grief that you might be experiencing pertaining to social relationships (Weissman, Markowitz, and Klerman 2000).

Several very effective psychological medications also might be effective for you, including such medications as tricyclic antidepressants, monoamine oxidase inhibitors, selective serotonin reuptake inhibitors (SSRIs), and atypical antidepressants such as buproprion and venlafaxine. Many of these medications have been effective in lessening feelings of depression and anxiety. In general, tricyclic antidepressants, SSRIs, and the newer atypical agents are the pharmacological treatments of choice. SSRIs and atypical antidepressants are generally preferred when effective because they have fewer and less problematic side effects.

For more severe depressions where other interventions have not been useful, other strategies such as electroconvulsive shock therapy or vagus nerve stimulation may provide some relief (Carpenter et al. 2006). Although the evidence is unclear at this stage, alternative treatments such as Saint-John's-wort and omega-3 fatty acids may also have promise as effective treatments for clinical depression.

Effectiveness of These Approaches

Research on the relative effectiveness of antidepressant medication and short-term psychotherapy in treating clinical depression has shown that both types of interventions can be successful. Importantly, a good body of work suggests that psychological and medication-based approaches generally are very comparable in reducing the symptoms of depression (DeRubeis and Crits-Christoph 1998; Hollon, Thase, and Markowitz 2002; Robinson, Berman, and Neimeyer

1990; Wolf and Hopko, in press). Some research suggests that in the short term, antidepressant medications may be more effective than interpersonal psychotherapy or cognitive behavioral therapy for individuals with less severe depression (Elkin et al. 1989). Other studies have suggested cognitive therapy is more effective than tricyclic medication in reducing depressive symptoms and in altering people's views of themselves, the world, and the future. Although a combined treatment might logically seem to be more effective than psychotherapy or medications alone, research has not yet demonstrated that multimodal therapy has a significant added benefit in treating clinical depression. However, several studies suggest this strategy may be promising among patients with more severe (chronic) depression (Keller et al. 2000). Importantly, there also are some data to suggest that depressed patients who respond to psychotherapy may be less likely to relapse following treatment termination compared with patients treated using only antidepressant medication (Hollon et al. 2002).

It has become evident that there are many factors that may be associated with a negative (or limited) treatment response to psychological and medication-based interventions. Among the factors that might limit the benefits of such approaches include increased severity and chronicity of depression, family history of depression, presence of a personality disorder such as borderline or histrionic personality disorder, coexistent anxiety disorders, perceived social stigma associated with being depressed, increased cognitive and/or social problems, marital discord, and reduced expectations that treatment will be successful (Hopko et al. 2004). Having one or several of these characteristics does not necessarily mean that you will have unsuccessful experiences using this workbook, being involved with therapy, or using various antidepressant medications. On the contrary, these are issues that you and possibly your mental health practitioner need to be aware of to assess whether or not you might require a more tailored and individualized intervention that will be most effective for you.

Moving Forward from Here

Congratulations on all you have accomplished in moving through this workbook. You are now fully equipped with the necessary skills to overcome your depression and anxiety. You have learned to better understand the relationships between the way you spend your time, your values and goals, and the level of avoidance in your life; how your mood is associated with how you behave; the difference between your present and ideal selves; and how to engage in behavioral activation to experience a more pleasurable and rewarding life that is characterized by less depression and anxiety. You have also learned effective strategies to better address issues with medication management and treatment, solve problems more effectively, get a better night's sleep, become more assertive and develop social skills, overcome your social anxiety, and learn how to feel more calm through the strategies of progressive muscle relaxation, mindfulness, and self-hypnosis.

Remember that as we discussed at the outset of this book, the race of working to overcome your depression and anxiety isn't about a sprint, nor is it necessarily about a marathon. Instead, the race that you have embarked upon is about making steady progress on the road toward psychological well-being. At times this road will be a very smooth one, marked by positive moods and a high sense of self-esteem. At other times, you will experience bumps on the road and bad weather that might slow you down on your travels toward mental health. When these obstacles come up, remember all the skills you have learned, the relapse-prevention strategies presented in this chapter, your commitment to change, and, once again, focus on incorporating these skills and abilities into your daily life. Also remember that you do not have to be controlled by your cancer, anxiety, or depression. Instead, take control of your life by focusing on what you have the power to change, namely the way you spend your time and how you behave on a daily basis. Do not avoid situations that might cause you fear or anxiety, and do not allow feelings of depression and anxiety to cause you to become a passive person in this world. Approach your problems, face your fears, and, even when feeling blue and depressed, do things that might cause you to feel a sense of pleasure or satisfaction despite these feelings. You can have a successful race and a productive, meaningful, and purpose-filled life. Our thoughts, prayers, and hopes are with you as you face the life challenges that will come your way.

Resources

NATIONAL CANCER ORGANIZATIONS AND RESOURCES

American Cancer Society
1599 Clifton Road, NE
Atlanta, Georgia, 30329-4251
(800) ACS-2345
www.cancer.org

Cancer Care
275 Seventh Avenue
New York, NY, 10001
(800) 813-4673
www.cancercare.org

Cancer Survivors Network
1201 16th Street NW
Suite 521
Washington, DC 20036
(877) 333-4673
www.acscsn.com

National Alliance of Breast Cancer Organizations
9 East 37th Street, 10th Floor
New York, NY 10016
(888) 806-2226
www.nabco.com

National Breast Cancer Coalition
1707 L Street, NW
Suite 1060
Washington, DC 20036
(202) 296-7477
www.natlbcc.org

National Cancer Institute
31 Center Drive, MCS 2580
Building 31, Room 10A31
Bethesda, MD 20892-2580
(800) 4-CANCER
www.nci.nih.gov

Susan G. Komen Alliance
Susan G. Komen Foundation
Occidental Tower
5005 LBJ Freeway, Suite 250
Dallas, TX 75224
(800) 462-9273
www.komen.org

American Institute for Cancer Research
1759 R Street
Washington, DC 20009
(800) 843-8114
www.aicr.org

References

Abramson, L. Y., G. I. Metalsky, and L. B. Alloy. 1989. Hopelessness depression: A theory-based subtype of depression. *Psychological Review* 96:358–72.

Addis, M. E., and C. R. Martell. 2004. *Overcoming Depression One Step at a Time: The New Behavioral Activation Approach for Getting Your Life Back.* Oakland, CA: New Harbinger Publications.

Akechi, T., T. Okuyama, N. Akizuki, K. Shimizu, M. Inagaki, M. Fujimori, Y. Shima, T. A. Furukawa, and Y. Uchitomi. 2006. Associated and predictive factors of sleep disturbance in advanced cancer patients. *Psycho-Oncology* 15:463–73.

American Cancer Society. 2005. *Cancer Facts and Figures.* American Cancer Society.

American Psychiatric Association. 2000. *Practice Guideline for the Treatment of Patients with Major Depressive Disorder,* 2nd ed. Arlington, VA: American Psychiatric Association.

American Psychiatric Association. 2001. *Diagnostic and Statistical Manual of Mental Disorders,* 4th ed. text revision. Washington, DC: American Psychiatric Association.

Anderson, K. O., C. J. Getto, T. R. Mendoza, S. N. Palmer, X. S. Wang, C. C. Reyes-Gibby, and C. S. Cleeland. 2003. Fatigue and sleep disturbance in patients with cancer, patients with clinical depression, and community-dwelling adults. *Journal of Pain and Symptom Management* 25:307–18.

Atkins. L., and L. Fallowfield. 2006. Intentional and non-intentional non-adherence to medication amongst breast cancer patients. *European Journal of Cancer* 42:2271–76.

Baer, R. A. 2003. Mindfulness training as a clinical intervention: A conceptual and empirical review. *Clinical Psychology: Science and Practice* 10:125–143.

Barlow, D. H. 2002. *Anxiety and Its Disorders: The Nature and Treatment of Anxiety and Panic,* 2nd ed. New York: Guilford.

Barlow, D. H., L. B. Allen, and M. L. Choate, 2004. Toward a unified treatment of emotional disorders. *Behavior Therapy* 35:205–30.

Baum, A., and B. L. Andersen. 2001. *Psychosocial Interventions for Cancer.* Washington, DC: American Psychological Association.

Beck, A. T., A. J. Rush, B. J. Shaw, and G. Emery. 1979. *Cognitive Therapy of Depression.* New York: Guilford Press.

Beckham, E. E., and W. R. Leber. 1995. *Handbook of Depression,* 2nd ed. New York: Guilford Press.

Berger, A. M., J. Sankaranarayanan, and S. Watanabe-Galloway. Forthcoming. Current methodological approaches to the study of sleep disturbances and quality of life in adults with cancer: a systematic review. *Psycho-Oncology.*

Brody, A. L., S. Saxena, P. Stoessel, L. A. Gillies, L. A. Fairbanks, S. Alborzian, M. E. Phelps, S. C. Huang, H. M. Wu, M. L. Ho, M. K. Ho, S. C. Au, K. Maidment, and L. R. Baxter. 2001. Regional brain metabolic changes in patients with major depression treated with either paroxetine or interpersonal therapy. *Archives of General Psychiatry* 58:631–40.

Brown, K. W., and R. M. Ryan. 2003. The benefits of being present: Mindfulness and its role in psychological well-being. *Journal of Personality and Social Psychology* 84:822–48.

Bruch, M. A., and R. G. Heimberg. 1994. Differences in perceptions of parental and personal characteristics between generalized and nongeneralized social phobics. *Journal of Anxiety Disorders* 8:155–68.

Carpenter, L. L., G. M. Friehs, A. R. Tyrka, S. Rasmussen, L. H. Price, and B. D. Greenberg. 2006. Vagus nerve stimulation and deep brain stimulation for treatment resistant depression. *Medicine and Health* 89:137–41.

Chambless, D. L., and T. H. Ollendick. 2001. Empirically supported psychological interventions: Controversies and evidence. *Annual Review of Psychology* 52:685–716.

Ciaramella, A., and P. Poli. 2001. Assessment of depression among cancer patients: The role of pain, cancer type, and treatment. *Psycho-Oncology* 10:156–65.

Cleeland, C.S., R. Gonin, A. K. Hatfield, J. H. Edmonson, R. H. Blum, J. A. Stewart, and K. J. Pandya. 1994. Pain and its treatment in patients with metastatic breast cancer. *New England Journal of Medicine* 9:592–96.

Craske, M. G. 2003. *Origins of Phobias and Anxiety Disorders: Why More Women Than Men?* Amsterdam: Elsevier.

Craske, M. G., D. H. Barlow, and T. A. O'Leary. 1992. *Mastery of Your Anxiety and Worry: Client Workbook.* New York: Graywind Publications Incorporated.

Croyle, R. T., and J. H. Rowland. 2003. Mood disorders and cancer: A National Cancer Institute perspective. *Biological Psychiatry* 54:191–94.

Davidson, J. R., A. W. MacLean, M. D. Brundage, and K. Schulze. 2002. Sleep disturbance in cancer patients. *Social Science and Medicine* 24:1309–21.

DeRubeis, R. J., and P. Crits-Christoph. 1998. Empirically-supported individual and group psychological treatments for adult mental disorders. *Journal of Consulting and Clinical Psychology* 66:37-52.

Dimidjian, S., S. Hollon, K. Dobson, K. Schmaling, B. Kohlenberg, M. E. Addis, R. Gallop, J. B. McGlinchey, D. K. Markley, J. K. Gollan, D. C. Atkins, D. L. Dunner, and N. S. Jacobson. 2006. Randomized trial of behavioral activation, cognitive therapy, and antidepressant medication in the acute treatment of adults with major depression. *Journal of Consulting and Clinical Psychology* 74:658-70.

Erblich, J., G. H. Montgomery, H. B. Valdimarsdottir, M. Cloitre, and D. H. Bovbjerg. 2003. Biased cognitive processing of cancer-related information among women with family histories of breast cancer: Evidence from a cancer Stroop task. *Health Psychology* 22:235-44.

Fernandes, R., P. Stone, P. Andrews, R. Morgan, and S. Sharma. 2006. Comparison between fatigue, sleep disturbance, and circadian rhythm in cancer inpatients and healthy volunteers: evaluation of diagnostic criteria for cancer-related fatigue. *Journal of Pain Symptom Management,* 32:245-54.

Flint, A. 1994. Epidemiology and comorbidity of anxiety in the elderly. *American Journal of Psychiatry* 151:640-49.

Frisch, M. B. 1999. Quality of life assessment/intervention and the Quality of Life Inventory (QOLI). In *The Use of Psychological Testing for Treatment Planning and Outcome Assessment,* 2nd ed. edited by M. E. Maruish. Mahwah, NJ: Erlbaum.

Gruzelier, J. 2002. A review of the impact of hypnosis, relaxation, guided imagery and individual differences on aspects of immunity and health. *Stress: The International Journal on the Biology of Stress* 5:147-63.

Gruzelier, J., A. Champion, P. Fox, M. Rollin, S. McCormack, P. Catalan, S. Barton, and D. Henderson. 2002. Individual differences in personality, immunology, and mood in patients undergoing self-hypnosis training for the successful treatment of a chronic viral illness, HSV-2. *Contemporary Hypnosis* 19:149-66.

Gruzelier, J., J. Levy, J. Williams, and D. Henderson. 2001. Self-hypnosis and exam stress: Comparing immune and relaxation-related imagery for influences on immunity, health, and mood. *Contemporary Hypnosis* 18:73-86.

Gruzelier, J., F. Smith, A. Nagy, and D. Henderson. 2001. Cellular and humoral immunity, mood and exam stress: The influences of self-hypnosis and personality predictors. *International Journal of Psychophysiology* 42:5-71.

Hawkins, R. M. F. 2001. A systematic meta-review of hypnosis as an empirically supported treatment for pain. *Pain Reviews* 8:47-73.

Hayes, S. C., K. D. Strosahl and K. G. Wilson. 1999. *Acceptance and Commitment Therapy: An Experiential Approach to Behavior Change.* New York: Guilford Press.

Hayes, S. C., K. W. Wilson, E. V. Gifford, V. M. Folette, and K. Strosahl. 1996. Experiential avoidance and behavioral disorders: A functional dimensional approach to diagnosis and treatment. *Journal of Clinical and Consulting Psychology* 64:1152-68.

Henderson, C. E. 2007. Self-hypnosis induction script. From: *www.bcx.net/hypnosis/script.htm* (accessed on 2/17/2007).

Hollon, S. D., M. E. Thase, and J. C. Markowitz. 2002. Treatment and prevention of depression. *Psychological Science in the Public Interest* 3:39-77.

Holmes, M. D., W. Y. Chen, D. Feskanich, C. H. Kroenke, and G. A. Colditz. 2005. Physical activity and survival after breast cancer diagnosis. *Journal of the American Medical Association* 293:2479-86.

Honda, K., and R. D. Goodwin. 2004. Cancer and mental disorders in a national community sample: Findings from the national comorbidity survey. *Psychotherapy and Psychosomatics* 73:235-42.

Hope, D. A., R. G. Heimberg, H. R. Juster, and C. L. Turk. 2000. *Managing Social Anxiety: A Cognitive-Behavioral Therapy Approach.* New York: Graywind Publications.

Hopko, D. R., J. L. Bell, M. E. A. Armento, M. K. Hunt, and C. W. Lejuez. 2005. Behavior therapy for depressed cancer patients in primary care. *Psychotherapy: Theory, Research, Practice, Training* 42:236-43.

Hopko, D. R., J. L. Bell, M. E. A. Armento, S. M. C. Robertson, C. Mullane, N. Wolf, and C. W. Lejuez. 2006. *CBATD for Depressed Cancer Patients in a Medical Care Setting.* Manuscript submitted for publication.

Hopko, D. R., S. D. Hopko, and C. W. Lejuez. 2004. Behavioral activation as an intervention for co-existent depressive and anxiety symptoms. *Clinical Case Studies* 3:37-48.

Hopko, D. R., C. W. Lejuez, M. E. A. Armento, and R. L. Bare. 2004. Depressive disorders. In *Psychological Assessment in Clinical Practice: A Pragmatic Guide,* edited by M. Hersen. New York: Taylor & Francis.

Hopko, D. R., C. W. Lejuez, J. LePage, S. D. Hopko, and D. W. McNeil. 2003. A brief behavioral activation treatment for depression: A randomized trial within an inpatient psychiatric hospital. *Behavior Modification* 27:458-69.

Hopko, D. R., and M. A. Stanley. 2003. Anxiety disorders in older adults: Assessment, treatment, and future directions. In *Directions in Clinical Counseling and Psychology.* New York: The Hatherleigh Company.

Howe, G. R., M. J. Friedenreich, M. Jain, and A. B. Miller. 1991. A cohort study of fat intake and risk of breast cancer. *Journal of the National Cancer Institute* 83:336-40.

International Agency for Research of Cancer. 1987. *IARC Monograph on the Evaluation of Carcinogenic Risks to Humans, Overall Evaluations of Carcinogenicity, Update of IARC Monograph.* Lyon, France: IARC.

Irwin, M., M. Fortner, C. Clark, J. McClintick, C. Costlow, J. White, S. Ancoli-Israel, and J. C. Gillin. 1995. Reduction of natural killer cell activity in primary insomnia and in major depression. *Sleep Research* 24:256.

Itano, J., P. Tanabe, J. L. Lum, L. Lamkin, E. Rizzo, M. Weiland, and P. Sata. 1983. Compliance of cancer patients to therapy. *Western Journal of Nursing Research* 5:5–20.

Jacobson, N. S., K. Dobson, P. A. Truax, M. E. Addis, K. Koerner. J. K. Gollan, E. Gortner, and S. E. Prince. 1996. A component analysis of cognitive-behavioral treatment for depression. *Journal of Consulting and Clinical Psychology* 64:295–304.

Jakupak, M., L. Roberts, C. Martell, P. Mulick, S. Michael, R. Reed, K. F. Balsam, D. Yoshimoto, and M. McFall. Forthcoming. A pilot study of behavioral activation for veterans with post-traumatic stress disorder. *Journal of Traumatic Stress.*

Kabat-Zinn, J. 1982. An outpatient program in behavioral medicine for chronic pain patients based on the practice of mindfulness meditation: Theoretical considerations and preliminary results. *General Hospital Psychiatry,* 4:33–47.

Kabat-Zinn, J. 2003. Mindfulness-based interventions in context: Past, present, and future. *Clinical Psychology: Science and Practice* 10:144–56.

Kabat-Zinn, J., M. D. Massion, J. Kristeller, L. G. Peterson, K. E. Fletcher, L. Pbert, W. R. Lenderking, and S. F. Santorelli. 1992. Effectiveness of a meditation-based stress reduction program in the treatment of anxiety disorders. *American Journal of Psychiatry* 149:936–43.

Kales, J. D., A. Kales, E. O. Bixler, C. R. Soldatos, R. J. Cadieux, G. J. Kashurba, and Vela-Bueno, A. 1984. Biopsychobehavioral correlates of insomnia: Clinical characteristics and behavioral correlates. *American Journal of Psychiatry* 141:1371–76.

Kangas, M., J. L. Henry, and R. A. Bryant. 2002. Post-traumatic stress disorder following cancer: A conceptual and empirical review. *Clinical Psychology Review* 22:499–524.

Kangas, M., J. L. Henry, and R. A. Bryant. 2005. The course of psychological disorders in the first year after cancer diagnosis. *Journal of Consulting and Clinical Psychology* 73:763–68.

Karacan, I., J. I. Thornby, A. M. Anch, G. H. Booth, R. L. Williams, and P. J. Salis. 1976. Dose related sleep disturbances induced by coffee and caffeine. *Clinical Pharmacology and Therapeutics* 20:682–89.

Kawachi, I., D. Sparrow, P. S. Vokonas, and S. T. Weiss.1994. Symptoms of anxiety and risk of coronary heart disease: The Normative Aging Study. *Circulation* 90:2225–29.

Keller, M. B., J. P. McCullough, D. N. Klein, B. Arnow, D. L. Dunner, A. J. Gelenberg, J. C. Markowitz, C. B. Nemeroff, J. M. Russell, M. E. Thase, M. H. Trivedi, and J. Zajecka. 2000. A comparison of nefazadone, the cognitive-behavioral analysis system of psychotherapy, and their combination for the treatment of chronic depression. *The New England Journal of Medicine* 342:1462–69.

Kessler, R. C., R. Avenevoli, and K. Ries-Merikangas. 2001. Mood disorders in children and adolescents: an epidemiologic perspective. *Biological Psychiatry* 49:1002-14.

Kessler, R. C., C. G. Davis, and K. S. Kendler. 1997. Childhood adversity and adult psychiatric disorder in the US National Comorbidity Survey. *Psychological Medicine* 27:1101–19.

Kessler, R. C., K. A. McGonagle, S. Zhao, C. B. Nelson, M. Hughes, S. Eshelman, H. U. Wittchen, and K. S. Kendler. 1994. Lifetime and 12-month prevalence of DSM-III-R psychiatric disorders in the United States. *Archives of General Psychiatry* 51:8–19.

Klerman, G. L., M. M. Weissman, B. J. Rounsaville and E. S. Chevron. 1984. *Interpersonal Psychotherapy of Depression.* New York: Basic Books.

Koster, E., E. Rassin, G. Crombez, and G. Naring. 2003. The paradoxical effects of suppressing anxious thoughts during imminent threat. *Behavior Therapy and Research* 42:1113–20.

Kristeller, J., and C. Hallett. 1999. An exploratory study of a meditation-based intervention for binge eating disorder. *Journal of Health Psychology* 4:357–63.

Laidlaw, T. M., and M. J. Willett. 2002. Self-hypnosis tapes for anxious cancer patients: An evaluation using Personalized Emotional Index (PEI) diary data. *Contemporary Hypnosis* 19:25–33.

Lee, K., M. Chow, C. Miaskowski, and M. Dodd. 2004. Impaired sleep and rhythms in people with cancer. *Sleep Medicine Review* 8:199–212.

Lejuez, C. W., D. R. Hopko, and S. D. Hopko. 2002. *The Brief Behavioral Activation Treatment for Depression (BATD): A Comprehensive Patient Guide.* Boston: Pearson Custom Publishing.

Linden, D. E. J. 2006. How psychotherapy changes the brain: The contribution of functional neuroimaging. *Molecular Psychiatry* 11:528–38.

Liossi, C., and P. White. 2001. Efficacy of clinical hypnosis in the enhancement of quality of life of terminally ill cancer patients: Erratum. *Contemporary Hypnosis* 18:220.

Lutgendorf, S. K., E. L. Johnsen, B. Cooper, B. Anderson, J. I. Sorosky, R. E. Buller, and K. Sood. 2002. Vascular endothelial growth factor and social support in patients with ovarian carcinoma. *Cancer* 95:808–15.

Lewinsohn, P. M. 1974. A behavioral approach to depression. In *The Psychology of Depression: Contemporary Theory and Research,* edited by R. M. Friedman and M. M. Katz, New York: Wiley.

Lewinsohn, P. M., I. H. Gotlib, M. Lewinsohn, J. R. Seely, and N. B. Allen. 1998. Gender differences in anxiety disorders and anxiety symptoms in adolescents. *Journal of Abnormal Psychology* 107:109–17.

Lyles, J. N., T. G. Burish, M.G. Krozely, and R. K. Oldham 1982. Efficacy of relaxation training and guided imagery in reducing the aversiveness of cancer chemotherapy. *Journal of Consulting and Clinical Psychology* 50:509–24.

Marcus, A. C., L. A. Crane, C. P. Kaplan, A. E. Reading, E. Savage, J. Gunning, G. Bernstein, and J. S. Berek. 1992. Improving adherence to screening follow-up among women with abnormal Pap smears: Results from a large clinic-based trial of three intervention strategies. *Medical Care* 30:216–30.

Martin, G., and J. Pear.1992. *Behavior Modification: What It Is and How to Do It,* 4th ed. Englewood Cliffs, New Jersey: Prentice Hall.

Martell, C. R., M. E. Addis, and N. S. Jacobson. 2001. *Depression in Context: Strategies for Guided Action.* New York: W. W. Norton.

Mazure, C. M., and G. P. Keita. 2006. *Understanding Depression in Women: Applying Empirical Research to Practice and Policy.* Washington, DC: American Psychological Association.

McGurk, R., L. Fallowfield, and Z. Winters. 2006. Information provision for patients by breast cancer teams about the side-effects of hormone treatments. *European Journal of Cancer* 42:1760-7.

McQuaid, J. R., M. B. Stein, C. Laffaye, and M. E. McCahill. 1999. Depression in a primary care clinic: The prevalence and impact of an unrecognized disorder. *Journal of Affective Disorders* 55:1–10.

Mineka, S., and R. Zinbarg. 1996. Conditioning and ethological models of anxiety disorders: Stress-in-dynamic-context anxiety models. In *Nebraska Symposium on Motivation,* edited by D. Hope. Lincoln: University of Nebraska Press.

Montgomery, G. H., K. N. DuHamel, and W. H. Redd. 2000. A meta-analysis of hypnotically-induced analgesia: How effective is hypnosis? *International Journal of Clinical and Experimental Hypnosis* 48:138–53.

Montgomery, G. H., C. R. Weltz, M. Seltz, and D. H. Bovbjerg. 2002. Brief presurgery hypnosis reduces distress and pain in excisional breast biopsy patients. *International Journal of Clinical and Experimental Hypnosis* 50:17–32.

Morin, C. M. 1993. *Insomnia: Psychological Assessment and Management.* New York: Guilford.

Mulick, P. S. and A. E. Naugle. 2004. Behavioral Activation for comorbid PTSD and major depression: A case study. *Cognitive and Behavioral Practice* 11:378–87.

Mynors-Wallis, L. 2005. *Problem-Solving Treatment for Anxiety and Depression: A Practical Guide.* Oxford: Oxford University Press.

National Cancer Institute. *www.cancer.gov.* Accessed 4/14/2007.

National Coalition for Cancer Survivorship. 2007. *www.canceradvocacy.org.* Accessed 4/13/2007.

National Institute of Mental Health 1995. Integration of Behavioral and Relaxation Approaches into the Treatment of Chronic Pain and Insomnia. NIH Technology Statement Online, 1-34. From *http://odp.od.nih.gov/consensus/ta/017/017statement.htm.* Accessed 4/13/2007.

National Sleep Foundation. *www.sleepfoundation.org.* Accessed 2/10/2007.

Newell, S. A., R. W. Sanson-Fisher, and N. J. Savolamin. 2002. Systematic review of psychological therapies for cancer patients: Overview and recommendations for future research. *Journal of the National Cancer Institute* 94:558–84.

Nezu, A. M. 1987. A problem-solving formulation of depression: A literature review and proposal of a pluristic model. *Clinical Psychology Review* 7:121–44.

Nezu, A. M. 2004. Problem solving and behavior therapy revisited. *Behavior Therapy* 35:1–33.

Nezu, A. M., C. M. Nezu, P. S. Houts, S. H. Friedman, and S. Faddis. 1999. Relevance of problem-solving therapy to psychosocial oncology. *Journal of Psychosocial Oncology* 16:5–26.

Nolen-Hoeksema, S., and J. S. Girgus. 1994. The emergence of gender differences in depression during adolescence. *Psychological Bulletin* 115:424–43.

Nolen-Hoeksema, S., and B. Jackson. 2001. Mediators of the gender difference in rumination. *Psychology of Women Quarterly* 25:37–47.

Ogden, J. 2004. *Health Psychology: A Textbook.* 3rd ed. Open University Press: Berkshire, England.

Palish, O. G., K. Collie, D. Batiuchok, J. Tilston, C. Koopman, M. L. Perlis, L. D. Butler, R. Carlson, and D. Spiegel. 2006. A longitudinal study of depression, pain, and stress as predictors of sleep disturbance among women with metastatic breast cancer. *Biological Psychology* 75:37–44.

Palmer, S. C., A. Kagee, J. C. Coyne, and A. DeMichele. 2004. Experience of trauma, distress, and post-traumatic stress disorder among breast cancer patients. *Psychosomatic Medicine* 66:258–64.

Patterson, D. R., and M.P. Jensen. 2003. Hypnosis and clinical pain. *Psychological Bulletin* 129:495–521.

Perlis, M. L., C. R. Jungquist, M. T. Smith, and D. Posner. 2004. *The Cognitive-Behavioral Treatment of Insomnia: A Treatment Manual.* New York: Springer.

Pigott, T. A. 1999. Gender differences in the epidemiology and treatment of anxiety disorders. *Journal of Clinical Psychiatry* 60:4–15.

Porter, J. F., C. Spates, and S. S. Smitham. 2004. Behavioral activation group therapy in public mental health settings: A pilot investigation. *Professional Psychology: Research & Practice* 35:297–301.

Purhonen, M., R. Kilpelainen-Less, A. Paakkonen, H. Ypparila, J. Lehtonen, and J. Karhu 2001. Effects of maternity on auditory event-related potentials to human sound. *Neuroreport* 17:2975–79.

Robinson, L. A., J. S. Berman, and R. A. Neimeyer. 1990. Psychotherapy for the treatment of depression: A comprehensive review of controlled outcome research. *Psychological Bulletin* 108:30–49.

Roemer, L., B. T. Litz, S. M. Orsillo, and A. W. Wagner. 2001. A preliminary investigation of the role of strategic withholding of emotions in PTSD. *Journal of Traumatic Stress* 14:143–50.

Savard, J., S. Simard, J. Blanchet, H. Ivers, and C. M. Morin. 2001. Prevalence, clinical characteristics, and risk factors for insomnia in the context of breast cancer. *Sleep* 24:583–90.

Segal, Z. V., J. M. G. Wiliams, and J. D. Teasdale. 2002. *Mindfulness-Based Cognitive Therapy for Depression: A New Approach to Preventing Relapse.* New York: Guilford Press.

Sheikh, J. I. 1992. Anxiety and its disorders in old age. In *Handbook of Mental Health and Aging,* 2nd ed., edited by J. E. Birren, R. B. Sloane, and G. D. Cohen. New York: Academic Press 410–32.

Singletary, S. E., and F. L. Greene. 2003. Revision of breast cancer staging: The sixth edition of the TNM classification. *Seminars in Surgical Oncology* 21:53–59.

Slaughter, J. R., A. Jain, S. Holmes, J. C. Reid, W. Bobo, and W. Sherrod. 2000. Panic disorder in hospitalized cancer patients. *Psycho-Oncology,* 9:253–58.

Smith, M. Y., W. H. Redd, C. Peyser, and D. Vogl. 1999. Post-traumatic stress disorder in cancer: A review. *Psycho-Oncology,* 8:421–37.

Soldatos, C. R., J. D. Kales, M. B. Scharf, E. O. Bixler, and A. Kales. 1980. Cigarette smoking associated with sleep difficulty. *Science* 207:551–53.

Speca, M., L. E. Carlson, E. Goodey, and M. Angen. 2000. A randomized, wait-list controlled clinical trial: The effect of a mindfulness-based stress reduction program on mood and symptoms of stress in cancer outpatients. *Psychosomatic Medicine* 62:613–22.

Spiegel, D., and J. R. Bloom. 1983. Group therapy and hypnosis reduce metastatic breast carcinoma pain. *Psychosomatic Medicine* 45:333–39.

Spiegel, D., J. R. Bloom, H. Kraemer, and E. Gottheil. 1989. Psychological support for cancer patients. *Lancet* 16:1447.

Spiegel, D., and J. Giese-Davis. 2003. Depression and cancer: Mechanisms and disease progression. *Biological Psychiatry* 54:269–82.

Stanley, M. A., G. Diefenbach, and D. R. Hopko. 2004. Cognitive-behavioral treatment for older adults with generalized anxiety disorder: A therapist manual for primary care settings. *Behavior Modification* 28:73–117.

Syrjala, K. L., G. W. Donaldson, M. W. Davis, M. E. Kippes, and J. E. Carr. 1995. Relaxation and imagery and cognitive-behavioral training reduce pain during cancer treatment: A controlled clinical trial. *Pain* 63:189–98.

Taenzer, P., R. Melzack, and M. E. Jeans. 1986. Influence of psychological factors on postoperative pain, mood, and analgesic requirements. *Pain* 24:331–42.

Teasdale, J. D., J. M. Williams, J. M. Soulsby, Z. V. Segal, V. A. Ridgeway, and M. A. Lau. 2000. Prevention of relapse and recurrence in major depression by mindfulness-based cognitive therapy. *Journal of Consulting and Clinical Psychology* 68:615–23.

Thase, M. E. 2006. Depression and sleep: Pathophysiology and treatment. *Dialogues in Clinical Neuroscience* 8:217–26.

Thase, M. E., J. B. Greenhouse, E. Frank, C. F. Reynolds, P. A. Pilkonis, K. Hurley, V. Grochoconski, and D. J. Kupfer. 1997. Treatment of major depression with psychotherapy or psychotherapy-pharmacotherapy combinations. *Archives of General Psychiatry* 54:989–91.

Theobald, D. E. 2004. Cancer pain, fatigue, distress, and insomnia in cancer patients. *Clinical Cornerstone* 6:15–21.

Turner, S. M., D. C. Beidel, and M. R. Cooley-Quille. 1997. *Social Effectiveness Therapy: A Therapist's Guide.* North Tonawanda, NY: Multi-Health Systems Inc.

Walker, L. G., S. D. Heys, and O. Eremin. 1999. Surviving cancer: Do psychosocial factors count? *Journal of Psychosomatic Research* 47:497–503.

Walker, L. G., M.B. Walker, and S. D. Heys. 1997. The psychological and psychiatric effects of rIL-2 therapy: A controlled clinical trial. *Psycho-Oncology* 6:290–301.

Walker, L. G., M. B. Walker, K. Ogston, S. D. Heys, A. K. Ah-See, I. D. Miller, A. W. Hutcheon, T. K. Sarkar, and O. Eremin. 1999. Psychological, clinical, and pathological effects of relaxation training and guided imagery during primary chemotherapy. *British Journal of Cancer* 80:262–68.

Weissman, M. M., J. C. Markowitz, and G. L. Klerman. 2000. *Comprehensive Guide to Interpersonal Psychotherapy.* New York: Basic Books.

Willett, W. C., M. J. Stampfer, G. A. Colditz, B. A. Rosner, and F. E. Speizer. 1990. Relation of meat, fat, and fiber intake to the risk of colon cancer in a prospective study among women. *New England Journal of Medicine* 323:1664–72.

Wolf, N., and D. R. Hopko. Forthcoming. Psychosocial and Pharmacological Interventions for Depressed Adults in Primary Care: A Critical Review. *Clinical Psychology Review.*

Wright, S., U. Courtney, and D. Crowther. 2002. A quantitative and qualitative pilot study of the perceived benefits of autogenic training for a group of people with cancer. *European Journal of Cancer Care* 11:122–30.

Zabora, J., K. Brintzenhofeszoc, B. Curbow, C. Hooker, and S. Piantadosi. 2001. The prevalence of distress by cancer site. *Psycho-Oncology* 10:19–28.

Zinbarg, R. E., and D. H. Barlow. 1991. Mixed anxiety-depression: A new diagnostic category? In *Chronic Anxiety: Generalized Anxiety Disorder and Mixed Anxiety-Depression,* edited by R. M. Rapee and D. H. Barlow. New York: Guilford.

Derek R. Hopko, Ph.D., is associate professor and associate department head in the Department of Psychology at the University of Tennessee. He graduated from West Virginia University and completed his residency and postdoctoral training at the University of Texas Medical School. His research and clinical interests focus on the behavioral assessment and treatment of mood and anxiety disorders. Hopko has strong interests in health psychology and conducts behavioral treatment outcome research with cancer patients diagnosed with clinical depression. He is a recipient of grant funding from the National Institute of Mental Health, the National Cancer Institute, and the Susan G. Komen Breast Cancer Foundation. He has authored some seventy peer-reviewed publications and serves on the editorial board of six journals.

Carl W. Lejuez, Ph.D., is associate professor in the Department of Psychology and founding director of the Center for Addictions, Personality, and Emotion Research (CAPER) at the University of Maryland. He graduated from West Virginia University and completed his clinical internship at Brown Medical School. Lejuez's current clinical and research interests focus on the treatment of mood and addictive disorders. He has published more than ninety-five articles and book chapters, served as principal investigator for more than ten grants from the National Institute of Drug Abuse, and has received Young Investigator Awards from the American Psychological Association Division of Experimental Psychology (Applied) and the Association for Behavioral and Cognitive Therapies (ABCT).

Foreword writer John L. Bell, MD, is professor of surgery and chief of the Division of Surgical Oncology at the University of Tennessee Graduate School of Medicine and director of the University of Tennessee Cancer Institute.

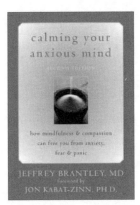
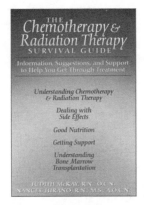
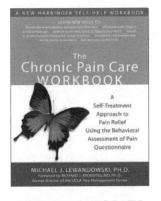
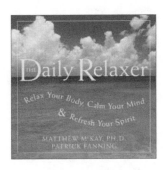
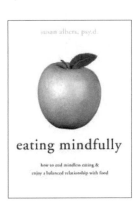
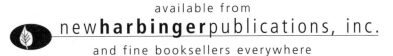

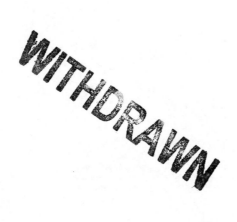